SCHEMA THERAPY MADE SIMPLE

Self-Help Strategies for Changing Core Beliefs

I0102938

Crystal Kita Logan

This book is intended to be a helpful resource for adults navigating late autism diagnosis. It represents the author's interpretation of current research and community knowledge at the time of writing. The field of autism research is rapidly evolving, and understanding continues to develop. Readers are encouraged to seek out the most current information and to connect with the autistic community for ongoing support and updated perspectives.

All case studies, examples, and personal stories presented in this book have been created as composite illustrations drawn from common experiences in the autistic community. Names, identifying details, and specific circumstances have been changed or combined to protect privacy and confidentiality. These examples are intended to illustrate typical challenges and experiences faced by late-diagnosed autistic adults but should not be taken as representing any specific individual's experience. Any resemblance to actual persons, living or dead, or actual events is purely coincidental.

ISBN: 978-1-7641438-9-9
Isohan Publishing

Table of Contents

Chapter 1: Meet Your Schemas (Core Beliefs) 1

Chapter 2: How Schemas Affect You Today......................12

Chapter 3: Where Did These Beliefs Come From? 24

Chapter 4: Healing Old Wounds..39

Chapter 5: Testing New Beliefs 56

Chapter 6: Daily Schema-Busting Techniques...................70

Chapter 7: Relationships and Schemas............................86

Chapter 8: Setbacks and Self-Compassion 98

Chapter 9: When to Seek Professional Help.....................111

Appendix A: Quick Reference Guides 125

Appendix B: Extended Exercises 141

Appendix C: Recommended Resources 151

Reference 159

Chapter 1: Meet Your Schemas (Core Beliefs)

Sarah stared at her phone, watching the three dots appear and disappear as Jake typed his message. Her heart raced, palms sweating. "We need to talk," finally appeared on the screen. She knew what came next—another relationship ending, another person leaving, another confirmation that she wasn't enough. This was her third breakup in two years, each following the same script: things start well, she becomes anxious about losing them, she clings tighter, and they pull away. Sarah didn't realize she was living out a pattern written decades ago in the neural pathways of her brain—a core belief system that whispered, "Everyone I love will eventually abandon me."

Opening Story: Sarah's Pattern

Sarah's story isn't unique. Like millions of people, she found herself trapped in repetitive life patterns that seemed to play on an endless loop. At 32, she had a successful career as a marketing director, owned her own condo, and maintained a circle of friends who genuinely cared about her. Yet in romantic relationships, she transformed into someone she barely recognized—needy, suspicious, constantly seeking reassurance.

The pattern started subtly. In the early weeks of dating, Sarah felt confident and secure. But as emotional intimacy grew, so did her anxiety. She'd check her phone obsessively, analyzing response times and emoji usage. If Jake took longer than usual to reply, her mind would spiral: "He's losing interest. He met someone else. I should have known this would happen." These thoughts felt like facts, not interpretations.

What Sarah didn't understand was that she was viewing every interaction through an invisible lens—one crafted in childhood when her father left the family when she was seven. Her eight-year-old brain, trying to make sense of the incomprehensible, had formed a belief: "People you love leave. You must have done something wrong." This belief, now hardwired into her adult brain, colored every romantic interaction like looking at the world through tinted glasses [1].

What Are Schemas?

Schemas are the mental "life rules" your brain created during childhood to help you survive and make sense of the world. Think of them as internal operating systems, quietly running in the background, influencing how you interpret situations, feel emotions, and make decisions. Jeffrey Young, who developed schema therapy, identified these as "broad, pervasive themes or patterns regarding oneself and one's relationship with others, developed during childhood or adolescence, elaborated throughout one's lifetime, and dysfunctional to a significant degree" [2].

Your brain is remarkably efficient. When you were young, it noticed patterns in your environment and relationships, then created shortcuts—schemas—to help you navigate similar situations quickly. If you grew up with an unpredictable parent, your brain might have developed a schema that says, "You can't trust people to be consistent." This protected you as a child by keeping you alert and prepared for sudden changes.

These schemas served a purpose—they were your brain's brilliant adaptation strategies. A child who develops a "self-reliance" schema after being repeatedly disappointed by caregivers learns to depend only on themselves. This might have been the smartest possible response to an unreliable environment. The problem arises when these outdated programs continue running in your adult life, in situations where they're no longer helpful or accurate [3].

The 18 Common Schemas with Friendly Names

Through decades of research and clinical work, psychologists have identified 18 core schemas that appear across cultures and backgrounds. Here they are with friendlier, more relatable names that capture their essence:

1. **"The Abandoned Child" (Abandonment/Instability)**: The deep fear that people you care about will leave, die, or emotionally withdraw from you.

2. **"The Mistrustful Detective" (Mistrust/Abuse)**: The expectation that others will hurt, humiliate, cheat, lie, manipulate, or take advantage of you.

3. **"The Lonely Island" (Emotional Deprivation)**: The belief that your needs for love, attention, and emotional support will never be adequately met.

4. **"The Flawed One" (Defectiveness/Shame)**: The feeling that you're fundamentally broken, bad, unwanted, or inferior in important ways.

5. **"The Outsider" (Social Isolation/Alienation)**: The sense that you're different from others and don't belong anywhere.

6. **"The Helpless Child" (Dependence/Incompetence)**: The belief that you can't handle daily responsibilities without considerable help from others.

7. **"The Sitting Duck" (Vulnerability to Harm)**: The exaggerated fear that catastrophe (medical, emotional, or external) could strike at any moment.

8. **"The Merged Identity" (Enmeshment)**: Excessive emotional involvement with important people, preventing individual identity development.

9. **"The Failed One" (Failure)**: The belief that you have failed, will inevitably fail, or are fundamentally inadequate compared to peers.

10. **"The Special One" (Entitlement/Grandiosity)**: The belief that you're superior to others and deserve special rights and privileges.

11. **"The Undisciplined One" (Insufficient Self-Control)**: Difficulty exercising self-control and frustration tolerance to achieve goals.

12. **"The People Pleaser" (Subjugation)**: Excessive surrendering of control to others to avoid anger, retaliation, or abandonment.

13. **"The Martyr" (Self-Sacrifice)**: Excessive focus on meeting others' needs at the expense of your own gratification.

14. **"The Approval Seeker" (Approval-Seeking)**: Excessive emphasis on gaining approval, recognition, or attention from others.

15. **"The Pessimist" (Negativity/Pessimism)**: A pervasive focus on the negative aspects of life while minimizing positive aspects.

16. **"The Controller" (Emotional Inhibition)**: Excessive inhibition of spontaneous action, feeling, or communication to avoid shame or loss of control.

17. **"The Perfectionist" (Unrelenting Standards)**: The belief that you must meet very high internalized standards to avoid criticism.

18. **"The Judge" (Punitiveness)**: The belief that people should be harshly punished for making mistakes.

Case Example 1: Marcus and "The Perfectionist"

Marcus, a 28-year-old software engineer, worked 70-hour weeks and still felt he wasn't doing enough. His code had to be flawless, his presentations perfect, his apartment spotless. When his manager praised his work, Marcus heard only the areas for improvement. "Your presentation was excellent, though next time you might want to add more visual aids," became "Your presentation wasn't good enough."

Growing up, Marcus's parents had high expectations. A 95% on a test prompted the question, "What happened to the other 5%?" They weren't cruel—they believed pushing Marcus would help him succeed. His child brain internalized this as "I must be perfect to be valued." Now, despite being promoted twice in three years, Marcus lived in constant fear of being exposed as incompetent [4].

Case Example 2: Elena and "The Abandoned Child"

Elena's abandonment schema manifested in friendships, not just romantic relationships. When her best friend Carmen started dating someone new and had less time for their weekly dinners, Elena's thoughts spiraled: "She's replacing me. I'm losing her. I should have known this would happen."

Elena's mother had died when she was five, and her father, overwhelmed with grief, had emotionally withdrawn. Various aunts and babysitters came and went. Elena's young brain concluded: "People leave when you need them most." Now at 35, she either clung too tightly to friendships or preemptively distanced herself to avoid the pain of eventual loss [5].

Case Example 3: David and "The Mistrustful Detective"

David approached every new relationship like a crime scene investigator. He analyzed text messages for hidden meanings, checked social media for signs of deception, and questioned motives behind kind gestures. When his colleague offered to help with a project, David thought, "What's his angle? He must want something."

David's schema developed after his older brother repeatedly borrowed his toys and broke them, then lied about it. His parents, busy with work, dismissed David's complaints as sibling squabbles. The eight-year-old David learned: "People will take advantage of you if you let your guard down." This protective mechanism served him then but now prevented him from forming genuine connections [6].

Quick Schema Identifier Quiz

Understanding which schemas influence your life is the first step toward change. This quick quiz helps identify your primary patterns. Answer yes or no to each question based on your gut reaction, not what you think you "should" answer.

For "The Abandoned Child":

1. Do you often worry that people close to you will leave or stop caring about you?

2. When someone is late or cancels plans, do you immediately think they're pulling away?

For "The Mistrustful Detective": 3. Do you often suspect others have hidden motives, even when they're being kind? 4. Is it hard for you to believe someone genuinely cares without wanting something in return?

For "The Lonely Island": 5. Do you feel like no one truly understands or "gets" you? 6. Even in relationships, do you often feel emotionally alone?

For "The Flawed One": 7. Do you fear that if people really knew you, they'd reject you? 8. Do you often feel fundamentally different from others in a bad way?

For "The Outsider": 9. Do you feel like you don't truly belong, even in groups where you're accepted? 10. Have you always felt like you're on the outside looking in?

For "The Helpless Child": 11. Do you often feel overwhelmed by everyday tasks that others seem to handle easily? 12. Do you frequently seek others' advice before making even small decisions?

For "The Sitting Duck": 13. Do you often worry about unlikely disasters (plane crashes, rare diseases, etc.)? 14. Does the world feel like a dangerous place where bad things are bound to happen?

For "The Merged Identity": 15. Is it hard to know where you end and your close relationships begin? 16. Do you feel guilty or anxious when you disagree with someone important to you?

For "The Failed One": 17. Do you feel like you're fundamentally less capable than your peers? 18. When you succeed, do you think it's luck rather than ability?

For "The Special One": 19. Do you often feel rules that apply to others shouldn't apply to you? 20. Do you get frustrated when people don't recognize your special qualities?

For "The Undisciplined One": 21. Do you often act on impulse and regret it later? 22. Is it hard to stick to goals when they require sustained effort?

For "The People Pleaser": 23. Do you regularly put others' needs before your own to keep peace? 24. Is it terrifying to think about someone being angry with you?

For "The Martyr": 25. Do you feel guilty when you do something just for yourself? 26. Do others often tell you that you give too much?

For "The Approval Seeker": 27. Does your self-worth drastically change based on others' opinions? 28. Do you change your behavior significantly depending on who you're with?

For "The Pessimist": 29. Do you automatically expect the worst in most situations? 30. When something good happens, do you immediately worry about what will go wrong?

For "The Controller": 31. Do you have trouble expressing emotions, even with close friends? 32. Do you fear losing control if you let yourself feel too much?

For "The Perfectionist": 33. Do you set standards for yourself that you'd never expect from others? 34. Is "good enough" never actually good enough for you?

For "The Judge": 35. Do you believe mistakes deserve harsh consequences? 36. Are you harder on yourself and others than most people seem to be?

Scoring Guide

Count your "yes" responses for each schema (questions are paired). If you answered yes to both questions for a schema, it's likely active in your life. If you answered yes to one question, it may be partially active. Most people have 3-5 schemas that significantly impact their lives, with 1-3 being primary drivers of their patterns.

Chapter Exercise: "My Top 3 Schemas" Worksheet

Now that you've completed the quiz, let's identify your top three schemas—the ones that most strongly influence your daily life.

Step 1: List Your Schemas Write down all schemas where you answered "yes" to both questions. These are your strongest patterns.

Step 2: Rank by Impact Consider which schemas:

- Cause you the most emotional pain

- Create the most problems in relationships

- Interfere most with your goals

- Come up most frequently in your thoughts

Step 3: Identify Your Top 3 Based on impact, select your three primary schemas. Write them here:

1. **Primary Schema:** _____ How it shows up in my life: _____

2. **Secondary Schema:** _____ How it shows up in my life: _____

3. **Third Schema:** _____ How it shows up in my life: _____

Step 4: Pattern Recognition For each of your top 3 schemas, write one specific example from the last month:

Schema 1 Example: _____ What happened: _____ How I interpreted it: _____ How I reacted:
_____

Schema 2 Example: _____ What happened: _____ How I interpreted it: _____ How I reacted:
_____

Schema 3 Example: _____ What happened: _____ How I interpreted it: _____ How I reacted:
_____

Key Takeaways

- **Schemas are childhood survival strategies** that helped you navigate early experiences but may no longer serve you

- **Everyone has schemas**—they're not character flaws but outdated mental programs

- **18 core schemas** have been identified, each representing a different core belief about yourself, others, or the world

- **Schemas influence** how you interpret situations, feel emotions, and behave in relationships

- **Identifying your schemas** is the first step toward changing patterns that no longer serve you

- **Multiple schemas** usually work together, creating complex patterns in your life

- **Awareness alone** doesn't change schemas, but it's the essential foundation for transformation

Your schemas aren't your fault—they're your brain's creative solutions to childhood challenges. Now that you can name and recognize them, you're ready to understand how they operate in your daily life. In the next chapter, we'll explore how these invisible beliefs shape your current experiences, reactions, and relationships, often without your conscious awareness.

Chapter 2: How Schemas Affect You Today

The coffee shop was crowded, but Emma barely noticed. Her attention was locked on her phone screen, where her friend Lisa's text sat unopened for the past hour. "Running late, be there in 20!" it read. For most people, this would be a minor inconvenience. For Emma, it triggered a cascade of thoughts and feelings that transformed her entire morning. Her chest tightened. Her mind raced: "She's always late when meeting me. She's probably with other friends. I'm not a priority. Maybe she doesn't even want to come." By the time Lisa arrived—exactly 20 minutes later as promised—Emma was cold, withdrawn, and barely responsive to Lisa's cheerful greeting. Lisa, confused by the chilly reception, became defensive. Their coffee date, meant to be a pleasant catch-up, devolved into awkward silence and hurt feelings on both sides.

The Schema Lens: How Core Beliefs Color Everything

Your schemas act like invisible filters, automatically interpreting every experience through their particular lens. Just as sunglasses tint everything you see, schemas color your perception of reality in predictable ways. The same event—a friend running late—gets processed completely differently depending on which schema is activated [7].

Let's examine how three different people with three different schemas might interpret the exact same situation: a friend canceling dinner plans at the last minute.

Through "The Abandoned Child" Lens (Abandonment Schema): When Michael receives the cancellation text, his abandonment schema immediately activates. His interpretation: "Here we go again. People always leave when I start counting on them. First it's dinner, next they'll stop responding to texts, then I'll lose another friend." His body responds as if he's experiencing actual abandonment—racing heart, sick feeling in his stomach, urge to either desperately reconnect or completely withdraw. He might send multiple texts seeking reassurance or delete the friend's number entirely, thinking, "Better to end it now than wait for the inevitable."

Through "The Flawed One" Lens (Defectiveness Schema): Sarah reads the same cancellation and her defectiveness schema springs into action. Her interpretation: "They must have realized spending time with me isn't worth it. I probably said something stupid last time we hung out. If I were more interesting/funnier/better, people wouldn't cancel on me." She feels a deep shame, a confirmation of what she "always knew"—that she's fundamentally not good enough. She might spend hours analyzing recent interactions, looking for evidence of where she went wrong.

Through "The Mistrustful Detective" Lens (Mistrust Schema): James gets the cancellation and his mistrust schema takes over. His interpretation: "They're lying about being sick. They probably got a better offer. People always have hidden agendas." He feels angry and vindicated—this proves what he's always suspected about people being dishonest. He might start checking social media to "catch" his friend in the lie or begin pulling away from the friendship, thinking he's protecting himself from further deception.

Notice how the same event—a friend canceling dinner—creates entirely different realities for each person. The friend might genuinely have the flu, but each schema creates its own story, complete with emotional reactions and behavioral responses [8].

Schema Triggers and Reactions

Understanding how schemas manifest in your body, emotions, and behavior helps you catch them in action. Schemas don't politely announce themselves; they hijack your entire system within milliseconds of being triggered.

Body Sensations: Your Early Warning System

Your body often knows a schema has been triggered before your conscious mind does. Each schema tends to create specific physical sensations:

- **Abandonment**: Hollow feeling in chest, like something is being pulled away; nausea; feeling physically cold

- **Defectiveness**: Heavy sensation, like carrying invisible weight; burning face; desire to physically hide

- **Mistrust**: Tension in jaw and shoulders; narrowed eyes; feeling physically on guard

- **Failure**: Sinking feeling in stomach; weakness in limbs; feeling physically small

- **Vulnerability**: Rapid heartbeat; sweaty palms; hypervigilance to physical sensations

Emma, from our opening example, experienced the classic abandonment response—chest tightening and a sick feeling—before her conscious thoughts even formed. These

14

body sensations aren't random; they're your nervous system preparing for what it perceives as a familiar threat [9].

Emotional Floods: When Feelings Overwhelm

Schemas trigger emotional responses that feel too big for the current situation. This disproportionate reaction is your first clue that you're responding to the past, not the present:

- **Sudden rage** over minor disappointments (entitlement schema activated)

- **Deep despair** from constructive feedback (failure schema activated)

- **Intense anxiety** from routine uncertainty (vulnerability schema activated)

- **Overwhelming loneliness** in a room full of people (emotional deprivation activated)

These emotions feel completely justified in the moment. Your schema has convinced you that this minor event is evidence of a major threat, so your emotional system responds accordingly [10].

Behavioral Patterns: The Schema's Endgame

Each schema drives specific behaviors designed to protect you from its feared outcome. Unfortunately, these protective behaviors often create the very situation you're trying to avoid:

- **Abandonment behaviors**: Clinging, constant reassurance-seeking, or preemptive rejection

- **Defectiveness behaviors**: Hiding authentic self, perfectionism, or self-sabotage

- **Mistrust behaviors**: Hypervigilance, testing people, or maintaining emotional distance
- **Subjugation behaviors**: Over-agreeing, suppressing needs, or chronic people-pleasing

The Schema Cycle (Illustrated Flowchart)

The schema cycle is a self-perpetuating loop that keeps you trapped in familiar patterns. Understanding this cycle is crucial for breaking free:

1. Trigger Event → 2. Schema Activation → 3. Automatic Interpretation → 4. Emotional Reaction → 5. Protective Behavior → 6. Consequence → 7. Schema Reinforcement

Let's follow this cycle with a detailed example:

1. Trigger Event: Your boss schedules an unexpected meeting

2. Schema Activation: Your failure schema switches on

3. Automatic Interpretation: "I must have messed up. They're going to fire me."

4. Emotional Reaction: Panic, shame, dread

5. Protective Behavior: You become defensive in the meeting, over-explain everything, appear anxious

6. Consequence: Your boss, who just wanted to discuss a new project, becomes concerned about your defensive behavior

7. Schema Reinforcement: You interpret their concern as confirmation you're failing, strengthening the schema

This cycle can complete itself in minutes, leaving you wondering why you keep ending up in the same situations [11].

Real-Life Examples

Case Example 1: Dating with an Abandonment Schema

Jessica, 29, had been dating Tom for four months. Things were going well—they laughed together, shared interests, and enjoyed each other's company. But as emotional intimacy grew, Jessica's abandonment schema became increasingly active.

The Trigger: Tom mentioned he'd be busy with a work project for the next two weeks and might not be able to see her as often.

Jessica's Internal Experience:

- Body: Immediate tightness in chest, cold sensation

- Thoughts: "This is how it starts. He's pulling away. Work is just an excuse."

- Emotions: Panic, desperation, profound loneliness

- Urge: To demand reassurance, to test his commitment

Jessica's Behaviors:

- Sent 15 texts in one day "just checking in"

- Suggested she could bring him dinner at work (he said no, he'd be in meetings)

- Interpreted his "K" response to a text as evidence of growing distance

- Showed up at his office with coffee "as a surprise"
- When he seemed stressed (about work), she assumed it was about her

The Outcome: Tom, feeling suffocated and confused by Jessica's sudden neediness, suggested they "slow things down." Jessica's worst fear—abandonment—became reality, not because Tom intended to leave, but because her schema-driven behaviors pushed him away.

The Reinforcement: Jessica thought, "I knew it. People always leave. I can sense these things. Good thing I saw it coming." Her abandonment schema grew stronger, ready to sabotage the next relationship [12].

Case Example 2: Work Life with a Failure Schema

Robert, 35, was a talented architect who consistently received positive performance reviews. Yet he lived in constant fear of being exposed as incompetent. His failure schema turned every workday into a minefield of potential humiliation.

Daily Triggers and Reactions:

- **Morning email check**: Seeing a meeting request made his stomach drop. "This is it. They've finally realized I don't know what I'm doing."
- **Presenting ideas**: He over-prepared to an exhausting degree, creating 50 slides when 10 would suffice. During presentations, he apologized preemptively: "This might not be perfect, but..."
- **Receiving feedback**: When his manager said, "Great work on the Johnson project. For the next one, let's

explore more modern materials," Robert heard only criticism. He worked until 2 AM researching modern materials, certain his job was at risk.

- **Team interactions**: When colleagues discussed projects without including him, he assumed they'd lost respect for his abilities, not considering they were simply working on different accounts.

The Pattern: Robert's schema made him work twice as hard as necessary, burning himself out trying to prevent a failure that existed only in his mind. Ironically, his exhaustion led to actual mistakes, which his schema interpreted as proof of his incompetence. When promoted to senior architect, Robert convinced himself it was a mistake or a diversity quota, not recognition of his genuine talent [13].

Case Example 3: Friendships with a Mistrust Schema

Ana, 31, longed for close friendships but found herself perpetually suspicious of others' motives. Her mistrust schema turned potential connections into investigations.

The Friendship Cycle:

- **Initial meeting**: Ana met Rachel at a book club. Rachel was warm and invited Ana for coffee.

- **Schema activation**: "Why is she being so nice? What does she want from me?"

- **Testing behaviors**: Ana mentioned fake plans to see if Rachel would gossip (she didn't). She "forgot" her wallet to see if Rachel expected payback for covering coffee (she didn't).

- **Partial trust**: After months of passed tests, Ana began to relax slightly.

- **The trigger**: Rachel couldn't attend Ana's birthday dinner due to a family obligation.

- **The interpretation**: "I knew it. She was just pretending to be my friend. The family thing is obviously a lie."

- **The investigation**: Ana checked Rachel's social media obsessively, looking for proof of deception. She found a photo of Rachel with her sister and interpreted Rachel's smile as "looking too happy for someone who supposedly had a family emergency."

- **The confrontation**: Ana sent a passive-aggressive text: "Hope your 'family emergency' worked out." Rachel, hurt and confused, responded with confusion.

- **The end**: The friendship dissolved, with Ana feeling vindicated: "I always know when people are lying."

Ana's mistrust schema created a self-fulfilling prophecy. Her suspicious behaviors and "tests" eventually pushed away genuine friends, confirming her belief that people can't be trusted [14].

Chapter Exercise: "My Schema in Action" Tracking Sheet

This exercise helps you recognize your schemas in real-time. For the next week, use this tracking sheet whenever you notice strong emotional reactions:

Date/Time: _____

Situation (Just the facts, like a camera would record):

Body Sensations (What did you feel physically?):

Automatic Thoughts (What immediately went through your mind?):

Emotions (Name all feelings and rate intensity 1-10):

My Behavior (What did you do or want to do?):

Which Schema Might Be Active? (Refer to your top 3 from Chapter 1):

Evidence For This Interpretation:

Evidence Against This Interpretation (This might be hard—try anyway):

Outcome (What actually happened?):

Reflection (How might the schema have influenced the outcome?):

Putting It All Together

Schemas don't just influence your life—they create your reality. They determine which aspects of a situation you notice, how you interpret ambiguous information, what emotions you feel, and how you respond. Like a film director who decides which scenes to include and which background music to play, your schemas craft the story of your daily experience.

The good news is that recognizing these patterns is the beginning of change. When you can say, "Oh, that's my abandonment schema talking," or "My failure schema is activated right now," you create a tiny space between trigger and response. In that space lies your freedom to choose differently.

Key Takeaways

- **Schemas act as invisible filters** that automatically interpret experiences according to their core beliefs

- **The same situation** triggers completely different reactions depending on which schema views it

- **Body sensations** often signal schema activation before conscious awareness

- **Emotional reactions** to schema triggers feel disproportionately intense for the current situation

- **Schema-driven behaviors** often create the very outcomes we're trying to avoid

- **The schema cycle** is self-reinforcing, using consequences as "proof" the schema is accurate

- **Multiple life areas** are affected—romantic relationships, friendships, work, and family dynamics

- **Tracking schemas in action** helps you recognize patterns and create space for different choices

- **Schema awareness** doesn't immediately change behavior but is essential for breaking patterns

Your schemas have been shaping your experiences for years, possibly decades. They've become so automatic that their influence feels like "just who you are." But schemas are learned patterns, not fixed personality traits. Understanding how they operate in your daily life is crucial preparation for the next step: exploring where these powerful beliefs came from in the first place. Once you understand their origins, you can begin to heal the wounds that created them.

Chapter 3: Where Did These Beliefs Come From?

Five-year-old Marcus sat at the dinner table, proudly showing his parents the picture he'd drawn at kindergarten. His teacher had put a gold star on it. "Look, Mommy! Mrs. Johnson said it was beautiful!" His mother glanced at the drawing—a house with a smiling sun—and pointed to the crooked chimney. "You need to work on making straight lines, sweetheart. And why is the sun wearing sunglasses? Suns don't wear sunglasses." His father added, "If you're going to do something, do it right. No one rewards mediocrity in the real world." Marcus's proud smile faded. He crumpled the drawing and threw it away after dinner. Twenty-three years later, Marcus would work until 3 AM perfecting a presentation, convinced that anything less than flawless meant failure.

Childhood Needs and Schema Formation

Every child enters the world with five core emotional needs. These aren't luxuries or preferences—they're psychological necessities as fundamental as food and shelter. When these needs are consistently met, children develop healthy beliefs about themselves, others, and the world. When they're not met, schemas form as protective adaptations [15].

The 5 Core Emotional Needs:

1. Secure Attachment and Safety Children need to feel safe, protected, and stably connected to caregivers. This includes:

- Predictable, nurturing responses to distress

- Protection from harm

- Consistent caregiver presence

- Emotional and physical safety

When met: Children develop trust, emotional security, and healthy attachment patterns. When unmet: Abandonment, mistrust, or vulnerability schemas may develop.

2. Autonomy, Competence, and Identity Children need opportunities to develop their own identity and confidence in their abilities:

- Age-appropriate independence

- Encouragement to explore and make mistakes

- Validation of their separate thoughts and feelings

- Support in developing personal capabilities

When met: Children develop confidence, self-reliance, and clear identity. When unmet: Dependence, failure, or enmeshment schemas may develop.

3. Freedom to Express Needs and Emotions Children need permission and safety to express their authentic feelings and needs:

- Acceptance of all emotions (not just "good" ones)

- Response to expressed needs

- Modeling of healthy emotional expression

- No punishment for having feelings

When met: Children develop emotional intelligence and healthy self-expression. When unmet: Subjugation, emotional deprivation, or emotional inhibition schemas may develop.

4. Spontaneity and Play Children need freedom to be children—to play, be silly, and act on impulse sometimes:

- Unstructured playtime
- Permission to be imperfect
- Joy and laughter in the home
- Balance between rules and freedom

When met: Children develop joy, creativity, and balanced self-control. When unmet: Unrelenting standards or insufficient self-control schemas may develop.

5. Realistic Limits and Self-Control Children need appropriate boundaries and guidance:

- Clear, consistent rules
- Age-appropriate expectations
- Teaching of consideration for others
- Balance between freedom and structure

When met: Children develop self-discipline and consideration for others. When unmet: Entitlement or insufficient self-control schemas may develop.

What Happens When Needs Aren't Met

When core needs go unmet, the child's brain doesn't simply accept this as unfortunate. Instead, it creates an explanation—a schema—that makes sense of the painful experience. These explanations generally fall into three categories:

1. **"It's my fault"** (I'm defective, I'm a failure, I'm bad)

2. **"It's how the world is"** (People leave, the world is dangerous, others can't be trusted)

3. **"It's what I must do"** (I must be perfect, I must please everyone, I must never need anything)

Young children are remarkably egocentric—not in a selfish way, but in believing they're the cause of everything around them. If daddy leaves, it must be because "I was bad." If mommy is always sad, it must be because "I'm not good enough to make her happy." These conclusions, formed by a child's limited understanding, become the schemas that guide adult life [16].

It's Not About Blame: Understanding Your Parents' Limitations

Before exploring schema origins, it's crucial to understand: This isn't about blaming parents or caregivers. Most parents do their best with the resources, knowledge, and emotional capacity they have. Many are struggling with their own schemas, passed down through generations like invisible family heirlooms.

Parents who can't meet their children's emotional needs often:

- Are dealing with their own trauma or mental health challenges

- Are overwhelmed by life circumstances (poverty, illness, loss)

- Are repeating patterns from their own childhoods

- Simply don't know better—parenting doesn't come with a manual

- Are doing much better than their own parents did

Understanding schema origins isn't about creating villains. It's about recognizing patterns with compassion—for yourself and for those who raised you. Your parents might have given you everything they had; it just might not have been everything you needed [17].

Common Schema Origins

Let's explore how specific childhood experiences tend to create particular schemas. These are patterns, not rules—every person's story is unique.

Abandonment Schema Origins

The abandonment schema typically develops from:

Actual Loss:

- Death of a parent or caregiver

- Parental divorce or separation

- Extended hospitalizations of child or parent

- Being given up for adoption

Emotional Abandonment:

- Caregiver depression or emotional unavailability

- Inconsistent caregiving (sometimes present, sometimes not)

- Threats of abandonment ("If you don't behave, I'm leaving")

- Frequent caregiver changes (multiple foster homes, nannies)

Seven-year-old Elena's mother died after a long illness. Her father, drowning in grief, sent her to live with different relatives every few months. Each time Elena began to attach to a new caregiver, she was moved again. Her child's mind concluded: "Everyone I love goes away. I must hold on tight or lose people."

Defectiveness Schema Origins

The defectiveness schema often stems from:

Direct Criticism:

- Constant criticism or comparison to others

- Being told you're "bad," "worthless," or "a mistake"

- Shame-based discipline ("You should be ashamed of yourself")

- Focus on flaws rather than strengths

Abuse or Rejection:

- Physical, sexual, or emotional abuse

- Bullying that goes unaddressed

- Being the "black sheep" or scapegoat in the family

- Rejection based on who you are (appearance, abilities, temperament)

Nine-year-old James was smaller than other boys and preferred reading to sports. His father, a former athlete, constantly expressed disappointment: "Why can't you be normal? What's wrong with you?" School bullies echoed this message. James concluded: "There's something fundamentally wrong with me."

Enmeshment Schema Origins

The enmeshment schema develops from:

Overprotective Parenting:

- Parents who won't let children take age-appropriate risks

- "Helicopter" parenting that prevents independence

- Messages that the world is too dangerous to navigate alone

- Doing everything for the child

Emotional Enmeshment:

- Being a parent's emotional support or "best friend"

- Having to manage a parent's emotions

- Guilt-tripping for normal independence ("How could you leave me?")

- No privacy or personal boundaries

Six-year-old Sofia's mother suffered from severe anxiety. Sofia learned to monitor her mother's moods, avoiding anything that might upset her. When Sofia wanted to play at friends' houses, her mother would cry: "You're all I have. Don't you love me?" Sofia concluded: "I'm responsible for others' feelings. My needs hurt people."

Case Example 1: The Making of a Perfectionist

Let's follow how Marcus (from our opening story) developed his unrelenting standards schema:

Age 5: The drawing incident. Marcus learns that his joy and pride can instantly turn to shame if his work isn't perfect.

Age 8: Report cards come home. Straight A's with one B+. Parents focus entire discussion on the B+. "We know you can do better." Marcus stays up past bedtime redoing homework until it's perfect.

Age 12: Makes the basketball team but isn't a starter. Father suggests maybe he should quit rather than "warm the bench." Marcus practices alone for hours every day until he injures his knee.

Age 16: Gets 1480 on SATs. Parents' response: "That's good, but Jake Henderson got 1540. Maybe you should retake it." Marcus signs up for expensive prep courses, studies constantly.

Age 20: In college, has a panic attack when he gets an A- on a paper. Begins taking stimulants to study longer. Professors praise his work; he only hears where it could improve.

The Schema's Birth: Marcus's developing brain, trying to earn his parents' approval and avoid their disappointment, created a rule: "I must be perfect to be valued. Anything less than perfect is failure." This wasn't conscious—it was a survival strategy for maintaining parental connection [18].

Case Example 2: The Birth of Abandonment

Elena's abandonment schema developed through layers of loss:

Age 5: Mother becomes ill. Hospital visits where mommy "looks different." Child's mind worries: "Did I make mommy sick?"

Age 6: Mother dies. Father cries constantly. Elena tries to comfort him but he pushes her away. "I can't right now, Elena."

Age 6-10: The relative shuffle begins:

- Aunt Maria (3 months): "I can't manage work and a child"

- Grandma (6 months): Has a stroke, can't care for Elena

- Aunt Sofia (4 months): Gets pregnant, "needs to focus on baby"

- Uncle Robert (5 months): Wife complains it's "too much"

Each Move's Impact:

- Elena learns not to unpack completely

- Stops calling caregivers "mom" or "dad" terms

- Becomes helpful and "easy" to avoid being sent away

- Develops stomachaches before each transition

The Schema Forms: Elena's brain creates an organizing principle: "People leave when you need them. Don't get too comfortable. Watch for signs of impending abandonment." By age 10, she's an expert at reading micro-expressions that might signal rejection [19].

Case Example 3: The Creation of Subjugation

David's subjugation schema arose from a household where his needs were consistently secondary:

Age 4: Little sister born premature, requires extensive care. David told repeatedly: "Be a good boy. Don't make trouble. Mommy needs to focus on the baby."

Age 7: Expresses anger about missing his birthday party for sister's medical appointment. Father's response: "How can you be so selfish? Your sister could die. Is your party more important than her life?"

Age 10: Wants to quit violin (which he hates) to play soccer. Mother cries: "I gave up my career for you kids. The least you can do is play the instrument I never could."

Age 13: Develops depression but doesn't tell anyone. Thinks: "They have enough to worry about with Sarah's health. My problems aren't that important."

The Pattern:

- David's feelings = selfish
- David's needs = burden
- David's job = make others' lives easier
- Good person = no needs

The Schema Crystallizes: David's brain develops a core belief: "My needs don't matter. Good people put everyone else first. Having needs makes me selfish and bad." This schema will guide his relationships for decades [20].

The Adaptive Child: Why These Beliefs Made Sense Then

Your schemas weren't thinking errors or character flaws— they were brilliant adaptations to challenging circumstances. The abandoned child who expects people to leave is trying to protect themselves from devastating surprise. The subjugated child who puts everyone first is maintaining crucial family connections. The perfectionist child is securing parental approval in the only way that seems to work.

Consider what would have happened if these children hadn't developed these strategies:

- If Elena hadn't learned to expect abandonment, each loss would have been freshly devastating

- If Marcus hadn't pursued perfection, he might have faced constant parental disappointment

- If David hadn't subjugated his needs, he might have been seen as another family burden

These schemas were psychological life rafts in rough seas. The problem isn't that you developed them—it's that you're still using them in calm waters, where they're no longer needed and actually prevent you from swimming freely [21].

Chapter Exercise: "Understanding My Story" Guided Reflection

This exercise helps you explore your schema origins with compassion and curiosity. Find a quiet space where you won't be interrupted.

Part 1: Childhood Needs Assessment

For each core need, reflect on your childhood experience (ages 0-12):

Secure Attachment and Safety

- Did you feel protected and safe most of the time?

- Were caregivers predictably available when you needed them?

- Could you count on emotional and physical safety?

- Rate how well this need was met: 1-10

Autonomy and Competence

- Were you encouraged to try things independently?

- Did caregivers believe in your abilities?

- Could you make age-appropriate choices?

- Rate how well this need was met: 1-10

Freedom to Express Needs and Emotions

- Were all your emotions acceptable (not just happy ones)?

- Could you express needs without punishment or shame?

- Did caregivers model healthy emotional expression?

- Rate how well this need was met: 1-10

Spontaneity and Play

- Was there joy and laughter in your home?

- Could you be silly and imperfect?

- Was there balance between rules and freedom?

- Rate how well this need was met: 1-10

Realistic Limits

- Were rules clear and consistent?
- Did you learn consideration for others?
- Were expectations age-appropriate?
- Rate how well this need was met: 1-10

Part 2: Connecting Needs to Schemas

Look at your lowest-rated needs. Which of your top 3 schemas might connect to these unmet needs?

Unmet Need: _____ Possible Connected Schema: _____ How they might connect: _____

Part 3: Your Origin Story

Choose one of your primary schemas. Write a brief, compassionate story about how it might have developed:

- What experiences contributed to this belief?
- How old were you when it started forming?
- How did this belief help you cope then?
- What would have happened if you hadn't developed this strategy?

Part 4: Compassion for All

Write a short paragraph of understanding for:

- Your child self who developed this schema
- Your caregivers who couldn't meet this need
- Your adult self who still carries this belief

Moving Forward with Compassion

Understanding where your schemas came from isn't about dwelling in the past or assigning blame. It's about recognizing that your core beliefs have a history—they're not ultimate truths about who you are or how the world works. They're outdated maps drawn by a child trying to navigate difficult terrain.

With this understanding, you can begin to:

- Recognize schemas as learned patterns, not fixed truths

- Have compassion for the child who needed these adaptations

- Understand that what protected you then may limit you now

- Begin imagining different beliefs that could guide your life

Your schemas have been with you for a long time. They've shaped your experiences, protected you from pain, and helped you survive. But survival isn't the same as thriving. Now that you understand where these beliefs came from, you're ready to begin healing the wounds that created them.

Key Takeaways

- **Five core emotional needs** must be met for healthy development: safety, autonomy, expression, play, and limits

- **Schemas form when needs go unmet**, as children create explanations for painful experiences

- **Children typically blame themselves** or create rules about the world to make sense of unmet needs

- **Parents' limitations** often stem from their own schemas, circumstances, or lack of knowledge

- **Specific experiences** tend to create predictable schemas, though each person's story is unique

- **Schemas were adaptive** in their original context—they helped children cope with difficult situations

- **Understanding origins** isn't about blame but about recognizing patterns with compassion

- **Your schemas protected you** when you needed protection; they're outdated strategies, not character flaws

- **Recognizing the child's logic** behind schemas helps separate past adaptations from present reality

In our next chapter, we'll begin the gentle work of healing these old wounds, meeting the needs of your inner child, and creating new, healthier beliefs to guide your adult life.

Chapter 4: Healing Old Wounds

Rebecca sat on her therapist's couch, arms crossed tightly across her chest. "I don't see the point in talking about my childhood," she said. "I'm 34 years old. What happened when I was six shouldn't matter anymore." Her therapist nodded gently. "You're right that you're not six anymore. But that six-year-old version of you is still in there, still hurting, still influencing your decisions. What if we could help her feel safe for the first time?" Rebecca's eyes filled with unexpected tears. She hadn't realized how much she'd been running from that scared little girl inside her—the one who still believed she was fundamentally unlovable.

Meeting Your Inner Child

The concept of an "inner child" might sound strange at first. You're an adult now, paying bills and making grown-up decisions. But neuroscience shows us that emotional memories from childhood remain remarkably intact in our brains, complete with the feelings, beliefs, and perspectives we had at that age [22]. When schemas get triggered, you're essentially experiencing the world through the eyes of your younger self.

Your inner child isn't just a metaphor—it's the emotional reality of your past experiences living within your adult self. This part of you holds both your wounds and your capacity for wonder, spontaneity, and healing. Meeting this younger version of yourself with compassion is the first step in healing schemas at their root.

Simple Guided Imagery Script

This exercise helps you connect with your inner child in a safe, controlled way. Read through it first, then close your eyes and guide yourself through it, or record yourself reading it slowly.

Preparation: Find a quiet, comfortable place where you won't be disturbed for 15-20 minutes. Sit comfortably with your feet on the floor.

The Journey:

Close your eyes and take three slow, deep breaths. With each exhale, let your body relax a little more.

In your mind's eye, see yourself walking down a gentle path. The path leads to a safe, beautiful place—maybe a garden, a cozy room, or a peaceful beach. This is your meeting place, and you have complete control over how it looks and feels.

As you explore this safe space, you notice a child in the distance. This child is you at a younger age—perhaps the age when your primary schema first formed. Notice what age they appear to be. Notice what they're wearing, their expression, their body language.

Approach slowly and gently. This younger you might be cautious or scared. That's okay. Sit down at a comfortable distance and simply be present. You might say, "Hi, I'm you when you're grown up. I came back to see you."

Notice how your younger self responds. They might come closer, or they might need more time. Let them lead. If they're willing, you might:

- Tell them they're safe now

- Let them know the difficult time will pass

- Share that you understand how hard things are

- Simply sit with them in quiet companionship

If your younger self wants to talk, listen. If they want to play, play. If they need to cry, let them know it's okay. You're not here to fix or rush anything—just to be present.

When it feels right (usually after 10-15 minutes), let your younger self know you'll come back. You might give them a hug if they want one, or simply wave goodbye. Know that this safe place exists whenever you need to return.

Slowly bring your attention back to your adult body. Feel your feet on the floor, your body in the chair. Take three deep breaths and open your eyes when ready.

Case Example 1: Sarah's First Meeting

Sarah, dealing with her abandonment schema, was skeptical about inner child work. "This feels silly," she thought. But she tried the visualization.

In her safe garden, she saw herself at age seven—the day her father left. Little Sarah was sitting alone on a swing, not swinging, just staring at the ground. Adult Sarah's heart broke. She approached slowly and sat on the grass nearby.

"I know Dad just left," Adult Sarah said softly. "And I know you think it's because you weren't good enough. But that's not true."

Little Sarah looked up, tears streaming. "Then why did he go?"

"Because he had his own problems that had nothing to do with you. You're loveable exactly as you are."

Little Sarah climbed into Adult Sarah's lap and sobbed. Adult Sarah held her, crying too, finally giving her younger self the comfort she'd needed for 25 years [23].

Drawing Exercise Option

Some people connect better through art than visualization. This alternative exercise can be especially powerful for those who struggle with mental imagery.

Materials needed: Paper and colored pencils, crayons, or markers (childhood art supplies often work best)

The Process:

1. With your non-dominant hand (to access a more childlike state), draw yourself as a child. Don't worry about artistic skill—stick figures are perfect.

2. Include details that feel important: What were you wearing? Where were you? What expression did you have?

3. Now, with your dominant hand, draw your adult self in the same picture. How are you positioned in relation to your child self?

4. Add any words, symbols, or colors that represent what you want to communicate between these two versions of you.

5. Look at your drawing. What do you notice? What does your inner child need from your adult self?

Case Example 2: Marcus's Drawing Discovery

Marcus, the perfectionist, resisted the "touchy-feely stuff" but agreed to try drawing. With his left hand, he drew a small stick figure hunched over a desk, surrounded by crumpled papers. The child had a frown and tears.

With his right hand, he drew his adult self standing behind the child. At first, Adult Marcus was holding a red pen, ready to correct. Then Marcus paused, erased the pen, and drew his adult self's hand on the child's shoulder instead. He added a speech bubble: "It's okay to make mistakes."

Looking at his drawing, Marcus was surprised by the emotion that welled up. He realized he'd internalized his parents' criticism so deeply that he'd become an even harsher critic of himself [24].

Reparenting Yourself

Reparenting is about giving yourself what you needed but didn't receive as a child. You can't change the past, but you can meet those needs now. This isn't about becoming your own parent in a literal sense—it's about taking responsibility for nurturing yourself in ways that heal old wounds.

What Your Younger Self Needed

Each schema points to specific unmet needs. Here's what the inner child behind each schema typically needs:

Abandonment: Consistent presence, reassurance of permanence, "I'm not going anywhere" **Mistrust**: Honesty, reliability, "I'll keep you safe" **Emotional Deprivation**: Attunement, understanding, "I see you and hear you" **Defectiveness**: Unconditional acceptance, "You're loveable exactly as you are" **Social Isolation**: Belonging, "You're one of us, you fit here" **Dependence**: Encouragement, belief in abilities, "You can do this, I believe in you" **Vulnerability**: Safety, protection, "I'll help you feel secure" **Enmeshment**:

Permission for autonomy, "It's okay to be yourself" **Failure**: Recognition of efforts, "I'm proud of you for trying" **Entitlement**: Balanced limits with love, "You're special AND others matter too" **Insufficient Self-Control**: Patient guidance, "Let's work on this together" **Subjugation**: Permission to have needs, "Your feelings matter" **Self-Sacrifice**: Modeling self-care, "It's good to take care of yourself" **Approval-Seeking**: Unconditional worth, "You're valuable just for being you" **Negativity**: Hope and reassurance, "Good things can happen" **Emotional Inhibition**: Permission to feel, "All your emotions are welcome" **Unrelenting Standards**: Permission to be human, "Good enough is good enough" **Punitiveness**: Compassion for mistakes, "Everyone makes mistakes, including you"

Giving Those Gifts to Yourself Now

Reparenting happens through consistent, small actions that meet your inner child's needs:

Daily Check-ins: Each morning, close your eyes and ask your inner child, "How are you feeling today? What do you need?" Listen without judgment.

Comfort Items: Keep objects that soothe your inner child— a soft blanket, a favorite tea, a childhood photo where you look happy.

Self-Soothing Practices: When triggered, use the soothing you needed as a child. Rock yourself gently, wrap yourself in a blanket, speak to yourself in a soft, kind voice.

Play Time: Schedule regular time for activities your inner child enjoys—coloring, swinging at a park, building with Legos, dancing to favorite songs.

Protective Boundaries: Be the protective parent you needed. Say no to people who treat you poorly. Leave situations that feel unsafe.

Celebrating Small Wins: Notice and celebrate your inner child's efforts, not just outcomes. "You tried something new today. That was brave!"

Daily Reparenting Practices

Here's a practical framework for daily reparenting:

Morning (5 minutes):

- Gentle wake-up (no harsh alarms)
- Kind words to yourself in the mirror
- Ask: "What does my inner child need today?"

Midday (2 minutes):

- Check in: "How am I doing?"
- One kind gesture to yourself
- Affirm: "I'm taking care of you"

Evening (5 minutes):

- Reflect: "What was hard today?"
- Comfort any difficult feelings
- Tuck yourself in with kindness

Weekend Ritual (30 minutes):

- Longer inner child connection
- Fun activity just for joy

- Create something without judgment

Case Example 3: Elena's Reparenting Journey

Elena, working on her abandonment schema, created a "permanence practice." Every morning, she looked in the mirror and said, "I'm here for you. I'm not going anywhere." She bought herself a locket with her own photo as a child, wearing it as a reminder of her commitment to herself.

When triggered by a friend canceling plans, she'd hold the locket and say, "I know this feels scary, like everyone leaves. But I'm still here. I'll always be here for you." She'd then do something nurturing—make her favorite childhood snack or watch a comforting movie.

Over months, Elena noticed the panicky feeling when people changed plans began to soften. Her inner child was starting to believe in her adult self's permanent presence [25].

The Compassionate Letter

Writing to your younger self externalizes the healing dialogue and creates a tangible reminder of your commitment to healing. This technique, drawn from compassion-focused therapy, helps solidify the reparenting relationship [26].

Template for Writing to Your Younger Self

Here's a structure to guide your letter:

Opening: "Dear [Your name] at age [age when schema was strong], I'm writing to you from the future, when you're [current age]..."

Acknowledgment: "I know right now you're experiencing [describe their situation]... I see how hard it is that [specific difficulty]... You're feeling [emotions] because [situation]..."

Validation: "It makes complete sense that you feel this way... Anyone in your situation would feel... You're doing the best you can with a really hard situation..."

Truth and Reassurance: "What you don't know yet is... The truth about the situation is... This difficult time will pass, and..."

Gifts and Promises: "I want you to know that... I promise to... You deserve..."

Closing: "I'm here for you always... With love and compassion, Your future self"

Examples from Different Schemas

Abandonment Schema Letter Excerpt: "Dear 7-year-old Emma, I know Daddy just left and you're scared Mommy might leave too. You keep being extra good, thinking if you're perfect enough, people will stay. Sweet girl, Daddy didn't leave because of anything you did or didn't do. Adults sometimes make choices that have nothing to do with children being good or bad. You could never be good enough to fix Daddy's problems, and you could never be bad enough to cause them. You're loveable exactly as you are—messy room, forgotten homework, temper tantrums and all..."

Defectiveness Schema Letter Excerpt: "Dear 10-year-old Marcus, I see you redoing your homework for the third time, erasing until the paper tears. Mom just said your drawing 'needs work,' and now you feel like YOU need work, like you're broken somehow. Beautiful boy, you're not a project to be fixed. You're a whole, complete person learning and growing. That drawing? It was creative and showed your unique way of seeing the world. Your worth isn't measured in perfect lines or grades or parents' approvals. You're valuable just for being you..."

Subjugation Schema Letter Excerpt: "Dear 8-year-old David, I see you giving your sister your favorite toy because she's sick again and everyone says you need to be 'the good big brother.' You wanted to play soccer but you're practicing violin because Mom gets that sad look when you mention quitting. Little one, your wants and needs matter too. Being good doesn't mean disappearing. You can care about others AND care about yourself. That's not selfish—that's healthy..."

Safe Place Visualization

Creating an internal sanctuary gives you a reliable retreat when schemas activate. This technique, used in EMDR and trauma therapy, provides emotional regulation and safety [27].

Creating an Internal Sanctuary

Your safe place should be:

- Completely under your control
- Free from any negative associations
- Filled with comfort and peace
- Accessible whenever needed

Building Your Sanctuary:

1. **Choose Your Space**: It might be:
   - A cozy cabin in the woods
   - A beach with perfect weather
   - A garden with high walls

- A library with endless books
- An imaginary floating island
- Your ideal bedroom

2. **Add Sensory Details**:
    - What do you see? (colors, light, objects)
    - What do you hear? (music, nature sounds, silence)
    - What do you smell? (flowers, ocean, baking bread)
    - What do you feel? (soft textures, warm sun, cool breeze)
    - What do you taste? (favorite foods available)

3. **Create Safety Features**:
    - Boundaries (walls, force fields, distance from others)
    - Comfort items (soft furniture, blankets, pillows)
    - Helpers (kind guides, protective animals, wise beings)
    - Control elements (you decide who can enter, ability to change anything)

4. **Practice Visiting**:
    - Start with 5-minute visits when calm
    - Notice how your body relaxes there

- Strengthen the visualization through repetition
- Add details each visit

When and How to Use It

Preventive Visits: Spend 5 minutes in your safe place each morning to start the day grounded.

During Trigger: When you notice schema activation:

1. Pause and breathe
2. Close your eyes (or soften your gaze)
3. Transport yourself to your safe place
4. Spend 2-3 minutes there
5. Return feeling more regulated

Before Difficult Situations: Visit your safe place before potentially triggering events (difficult conversations, social situations, work presentations).

For Sleep: A modified version can help with schema-related sleep issues—imagine yourself resting peacefully in your sanctuary.

Chapter Exercises

"Letter to Little Me" Template

Use this fill-in template to write your own compassionate letter:

Dear _____ at age _____,

I'm writing to you from the future, when you're _____ years old and you've learned so much about yourself and the world.

I know right now you're experiencing

_____

I see how hard it is that

_____

You're feeling _____ because

_____

It makes complete sense that you feel this way. Anyone who
_____ _____ would feel
_____

What you don't know yet is

_____

The truth about this situation is

_____

I want you to know that you are

_____

You deserve

_____

I promise to

_____

_____

Even though things are hard right now,

_____

_____

I'm here for you always. I'll never leave you or judge you or stop caring about you.

With endless love and compassion, Your future self

(_____)

"My Reparenting Plan" Worksheet

Create your personalized reparenting practice:

My Inner Child's Age: _____

Their Primary Need:

_____

Daily Reparenting Rituals: Morning:

_____

Midday:

_____

Evening:

_____

Weekly Special Time: Activity:

_____

When:

_____

—

Comfort Kit (5 items that soothe my inner child):

1. _____
2. _____
3. _____
4. _____
5. _____

My Reparenting Affirmations (3 phrases my inner child needs to hear):

1. _____
2. _____
3. _____

Signs of Progress (How I'll know the reparenting is working):

_____

_____

Commitment Statement: I commit to showing up for my inner child by _____

_____

Signed: _____ Date: _____

The Journey Forward

Healing old wounds isn't about erasing the past or pretending difficult things didn't happen. It's about changing your relationship with those experiences. Your inner child has been waiting—sometimes for decades—for someone to truly see their pain, validate their experience, and provide the comfort they needed.

That someone is you. Not the you who was also struggling and surviving, but the you who has grown, learned, and developed resources your younger self couldn't imagine. You have become the adult your inner child needed.

This work takes courage. Meeting your younger self means feeling old pain. But it also means finally giving that part of you what they've always needed—understanding, compassion, and unconditional love. With consistent practice, the scared, hurt, or lonely child inside begins to trust that they're truly safe now.

Key Takeaways

- **Your inner child** is the emotional reality of your younger self, still active in your adult life

- **Meeting your inner child** through visualization or drawing creates connection with wounded parts

- **Each schema** points to specific childhood needs that went unmet

- **Reparenting yourself** means actively providing what your younger self needed but didn't receive

- **Daily reparenting practices** build new neural pathways of self-compassion and care

- **Compassionate letters** externalize healing dialogue and create tangible reminders of commitment

- **A safe place visualization** provides an always-available internal sanctuary for emotional regulation

- **Healing happens** through consistent small actions, not one dramatic breakthrough

- **You can become** the caring, protective adult your inner child always needed

As you practice these healing techniques, you're literally rewiring your brain, creating new patterns of self-relationship. But healing is just the beginning. Next, we'll explore how to test new beliefs in the real world, gathering evidence that challenges the old schemas your inner child developed for protection.

Chapter 5: Testing New Beliefs

Dr. Martinez stood before her psychology class, holding two pairs of glasses. "These," she said, putting on dark sunglasses, "are like our schemas. They color everything we see. If I wear these all day, I'll think the world is darker than it really is." She switched to clear lenses. "Healing work helps us see our schemas. But to truly change, we need to test reality without them." She invited a student to describe what they saw through each pair. "The room didn't change," the student realized. "Just how I saw it." Dr. Martinez smiled. "Exactly. Your next assignment is to become scientists of your own lives—testing whether your core beliefs match reality or just feel true because you've worn those lenses for so long."

The Scientist Approach

You've spent years gathering evidence that supports your schemas. Every time someone left (abandonment), every criticism (defectiveness), every disappointment (failure) got filed away as proof that your core beliefs were accurate. But here's what your schema never told you: you've been conducting biased research.

Think about how a detective who's already decided who's guilty might investigate a crime. They'd notice every clue supporting their theory while overlooking evidence pointing elsewhere. Your schemas have made you a biased detective in your own life, collecting only evidence that confirms what you already believe [28].

The scientist approach means treating your beliefs as hypotheses—not facts—and testing them with genuine curiosity about what you'll discover.

Your Beliefs as Hypotheses to Test

In science, a hypothesis is an educated guess that needs testing. Your schemas are hypotheses about how the world works, formed by a child trying to make sense of difficult experiences. Now it's time to test whether these hypotheses hold up to adult scrutiny.

Transforming Schemas into Testable Hypotheses:

- **Schema**: "I'm defective" **Hypothesis**: "If people really know me, they'll reject me" **Test**: Share something genuine with someone safe and observe their response

- **Schema**: "People always leave" **Hypothesis**: "Close relationships always end in abandonment" **Test**: Notice relationships that have lasted, looking for disconfirming evidence

- **Schema**: "I must be perfect" **Hypothesis**: "Making mistakes leads to catastrophic consequences" **Test**: Deliberately make a small mistake and document what actually happens

Gathering Evidence Fairly

Fair evidence gathering means:

1. **Looking for disconfirming evidence** (what contradicts your schema)

2. **Considering alternative explanations** for events

3. **Checking your interpretations** with trusted others

4. **Recording actual outcomes**, not feared ones

5. **Noticing the middle ground** between extremes

Case Example 1: Jennifer's Mistrust Experiment

Jennifer, 33, believed "People only act nice when they want something." Her therapist helped her design an experiment:

Hypothesis: "The barista is only friendly because she wants a tip"

Experiment: Go to the same coffee shop for two weeks. Week 1: Tip normally. Week 2: Don't tip. Record the barista's friendliness level.

Jennifer's Prediction: "She'll be cold and rude when I stop tipping"

Actual Results:

- Week 1: Barista smiled, asked about her day, remembered her order

- Week 2: Barista still smiled, still asked about her day, still remembered her order

- Only difference: No "Have a great day!" on two occasions, but she seemed rushed those times

Jennifer's Learning: "She was consistently kind regardless of tips. Maybe some people are just... nice?" This small crack in her mistrust schema led to bigger experiments with trusting friends [29].

Behavioral Experiments Table

Here are 10 detailed examples across different schemas, showing the complete experimental process:

1. Abandonment Schema Experiment

- **Old Belief**: "If I'm not constantly available, people will replace me"
- **Prediction**: "If I don't respond to texts immediately, friends will stop including me"
- **New Behavior**: Wait 2-4 hours before responding to non-urgent texts
- **Actual Outcome**: Friends continued texting. One said, "It's nice you're not always on your phone anymore"

2. Defectiveness Schema Experiment

- **Old Belief**: "If people see the real me, they'll be disgusted"
- **Prediction**: "If I share my struggle with anxiety, my coworker will think I'm weak"
- **New Behavior**: Tell one trusted coworker about anxiety during lunch
- **Actual Outcome**: Coworker shared their own therapy experience, bonding deepened

3. Failure Schema Experiment

- **Old Belief**: "I'm incompetent compared to others"
- **Prediction**: "If I volunteer to lead the project, everyone will see I don't know what I'm doing"
- **New Behavior**: Volunteer to lead a small team project
- **Actual Outcome**: Project went well, team appreciated leadership, boss gave positive feedback

4. Emotional Deprivation Schema Experiment

- **Old Belief**: "No one really cares about my feelings"

- **Prediction**: "If I tell my friend I'm sad, they'll change the subject"

- **New Behavior**: Share feeling sad about something specific with a close friend

- **Actual Outcome**: Friend listened for 30 minutes, offered support, checked in the next day

5. Subjugation Schema Experiment

- **Old Belief**: "My needs don't matter"

- **Prediction**: "If I say no to overtime, my boss will be furious"

- **New Behavior**: Politely decline non-emergency weekend work once

- **Actual Outcome**: Boss said "Okay, see you Monday," assigned task to someone else

6. Unrelenting Standards Schema Experiment

- **Old Belief**: "Anything less than perfect is failure"

- **Prediction**: "If I submit a 'good enough' report, I'll be criticized harshly"

- **New Behavior**: Submit a solid B+ report instead of staying late to make it A+

- **Actual Outcome**: Report accepted without comment, saved 3 hours of work

7. Entitlement Schema Experiment

- **Old Belief**: "Rules don't apply to me"

- **Prediction**: "Waiting in line like everyone else is beneath me"

- **New Behavior**: Wait in full queue without trying to skip or complain

- **Actual Outcome**: Nothing bad happened, had pleasant chat with another person waiting

8. Social Isolation Schema Experiment

- **Old Belief**: "I don't fit in anywhere"

- **Prediction**: "If I join the book club, I'll have nothing to contribute"

- **New Behavior**: Attend book club and share one opinion

- **Actual Outcome**: Others agreed with perspective, invited to coffee after

9. Vulnerability Schema Experiment

- **Old Belief**: "Catastrophe could strike any moment"

- **Prediction**: "If I don't check the stove 5 times, the house will burn down"

- **New Behavior**: Check stove only once before leaving

- **Actual Outcome**: Anxiety initially high, house fine, anxiety decreased over time

10. Emotional Inhibition Schema Experiment

- **Old Belief**: "Showing emotions is dangerous"

- **Prediction**: "If I laugh loudly at the movies, people will judge me"
- **New Behavior**: Allow natural laughter during funny movie scene
- **Actual Outcome**: Others laughed too, one person said "Great laugh!"

Blank Behavioral Experiment Template

Use this template to design your own experiments:

My Schema:

_____

Old Belief:

_____

Specific Prediction:

_____ (What exactly do

I think will happen?)

New Behavior to Test:

_____ (What will I do

differently?)

When/Where I'll Test This:

_____

What Actually Happened:

_____

What This Tells Me:

_____

Starting Small The 10% Rule

The biggest mistake people make is trying to change too much too fast. If your abandonment schema has you texting partners 50 times a day, dropping to 5 texts immediately will trigger overwhelming anxiety. Instead, use the 10% rule.

Tiny Changes That Don't Trigger Overwhelm

The 10% rule means changing your behavior by just 10% from baseline:

- **Instead of** checking partner's social media 20 times → check 18 times

- **Instead of** saying yes to everything → say "Let me think about it" once

- **Instead of** redoing work 5 times → redo it 4 times

- **Instead of** avoiding all social events → attend for 10 minutes

These tiny changes fly under your schema's radar. Your protective system doesn't activate full alarm mode because the change seems insignificant. But these small shifts create proof that nothing terrible happens when you loosen your schema's rules.

Building Confidence Gradually

Each successful tiny experiment builds evidence and confidence for slightly bigger ones:

Week 1: Reduce checking behaviors by 10% **Week 2**: If anxiety was manageable, reduce by another 10% **Week 3**: Continue if ready, or stay at Week 2 level longer **Week 4**: Notice patterns, celebrate small wins

The goal isn't to eliminate all schema-driven behaviors immediately. It's to prove to your nervous system that loosening the schema's grip is safe.

Case Example 2: Tom's Perfectionism Steps

Tom's unrelenting standards had him rewriting emails dozens of times. His experiment ladder:

Week 1: Send one internal email after only 5 rewrites instead of 10 **Week 2**: Send two internal emails after 5 rewrites **Week 3**: Send one email after 3 rewrites **Week 4**: Send quick "Thanks!" emails without rewriting **Week 8**: Send important email after 2 rewrites **Week 12**: Send most emails after one proofread

"I couldn't believe it," Tom reported. "No one noticed. No disasters. My anxiety went from 9/10 to maybe 3/10 for regular emails. I still polish important ones, but I've reclaimed hours each week" [30].

Common Obstacles and Solutions

Testing new beliefs isn't smooth sailing. Here are the most common obstacles and how to navigate them:

"But What If It Goes Badly?"

Your schema will catastrophize about experiments. Common fears and reality checks:

Fear: "If I speak up in the meeting, I'll be fired" **Reality Check**: When was the last time someone was fired for contributing ideas? **Solution**: Start with lower-stakes situations—speak up with friends before important meetings

Fear: "If I don't triple-check my work, I'll make a horrible mistake" **Reality Check**: How many horrible mistakes have you made despite all that checking? **Solution**: Check twice instead of three times first, build from there

Fear: "If I show vulnerability, I'll be attacked" **Reality Check**: Test with safe people first, not your harshest critic **Solution**: Share something slightly vulnerable, not your deepest secret

Dealing with Setbacks

Sometimes experiments don't go as hoped. This doesn't mean your schema is right—it means you're learning.

Common Setbacks:

1. **The Self-Fulfilling Prophecy**: Your anxiety about the experiment influences the outcome

    o *Solution*: Notice and record your anxiety level, try again when calmer

2. **Picking the Wrong Person/Situation**: Testing trust with someone untrustworthy

    o *Solution*: Be more selective about experimental conditions

3. **All-or-Nothing Interpretation**: One negative result "proves" schema is true

    o *Solution*: Run 10 experiments before drawing conclusions

4. **Schema Hijacking**: Mid-experiment, schema takes over and sabotages

    ◦   *Solution*: Plan for this, have coping strategies ready

Case Example 3: Maria's Setback Learning

Maria, testing her defectiveness schema, shared a personal story with a coworker who responded awkwardly and changed the subject. "See?" her schema declared. "You're too much. People can't handle the real you."

But Maria's therapist helped her analyze:

- The coworker had just received bad news that morning

- Maria shared at a busy, public moment

- The coworker later apologized, saying "Sorry I was distracted earlier"

Maria's learning: "The experiment design matters. Timing, setting, and the other person's state affect outcomes. This wasn't about my defectiveness" [31].

The Progress Spiral (Not Linear)

Progress in challenging schemas follows a spiral pattern, not a straight line:

Better experiments

↗   ↘

Confidence Setback

↖ ↙

Learning & Adjusting

You'll circle through the same issues but at higher levels each time. The abandonment fears that once paralyzed you might still whisper, but now you respond differently. This isn't failure—it's the natural pattern of growth.

Signs of Spiral Progress:

- Faster recovery from setbacks

- Less anxiety during experiments

- Natural behavior changes without forcing

- Catching schemas earlier

- Compassion for the process

Chapter Exercise "My First Three Experiments" Planning Sheet

Design three experiments, starting with the easiest:

Experiment 1 (Easiest) Schema to Test:
_____ Old
Belief: _____
New Behavior (10% change):
_____ When I'll Try This:
_____ Support I Might
Need: _____

Experiment 2 (Medium) Schema to Test:
_____ Old
Belief: _____
New Behavior:
_____ When
I'll Try This: _____
What I Learned from Experiment 1 to Apply:
_____

Experiment 3 (Stretch) Schema to Test:

_____ Old

Belief: _____

New Behavior:

_____ When

I'll Try This: _____

How I'll Celebrate Courage Regardless of Outcome:

_____

Accountability Plan: Who I'll Share My Experiments With:

_____ How I'll Track Results:

_____ What I'll Do If I

Get Overwhelmed: _____

The Evidence Mounts

Every behavioral experiment is a vote for a new way of being. You're not trying to prove your schemas wrong through logic—they don't respond to logic. You're accumulating lived experience that contradicts their dire predictions.

Some experiments will confirm aspects of your schemas. Yes, some people do leave. Yes, rejection happens. Yes, mistakes have consequences. But experiments reveal the whole truth: not everyone leaves, not all mistakes are catastrophic, not every vulnerability leads to attack.

Your schemas show you a world painted in absolutes—always, never, everyone, no one. Experiments reveal the real world painted in nuance—sometimes, often, some people, in certain circumstances. This nuanced view gives you choice. You can respond to actual present-moment circumstances rather than reacting to schema-filtered distortions.

Key Takeaways

- **Schemas act like biased detectives**, collecting only evidence that confirms existing beliefs

- **The scientist approach** treats beliefs as hypotheses to test, not facts to defend

- **Behavioral experiments** test schema predictions against reality in controlled ways

- **Fair evidence gathering** means looking for disconfirming evidence and alternative explanations

- **The 10% rule** creates tiny changes that don't trigger overwhelming schema activation

- **Setbacks are learning opportunities**, not proof that schemas are correct

- **Progress follows a spiral pattern**, revisiting issues at increasingly higher levels

- **Small experiments build evidence** that the world is safer than schemas suggest

- **Success is in the courage to test**, not in perfect outcomes

You've been living by rules written by a child in distress. Through experiments, you're discovering which rules still serve you and which ones you've outgrown. This evidence forms the foundation for lasting change. But change requires daily practice. In our next chapter, we'll explore practical techniques to reinforce your new beliefs every single day.

Chapter 6: Daily Schema-Busting Techniques

The alarm went off at 6:30 AM, and immediately David's mind began its familiar script: "Another day to fail. I should have prepared more for that presentation. Everyone will see I don't belong here." For twenty years, David had started each morning marinating in self-criticism, setting the tone for days filled with anxiety and self-doubt. But this morning was different. David reached for his phone, not to check emails that would fuel his failure schema, but to play a two-minute recording he'd made: "Good morning, David. You're starting fresh today. You've prepared well. You belong here as much as anyone. Let's see what good things unfold." It felt awkward, almost silly. But by the time he'd finished his new morning routine—affirmation, brief meditation, and setting one kind intention for himself—David noticed something shift. The day ahead felt less like a minefield and more like an opportunity.

Morning Practices

How you start your day sets the neural pathways for everything that follows. Schemas love to hijack your barely-conscious morning mind, filling it with their predictions of doom, abandonment, or failure before you've even had coffee. Taking charge of your morning means choosing which voice gets to speak first.

Schema-Specific Affirmations

Affirmations work best when they directly counter your specific schema's lies. Generic positive thinking bounces off schemas like rain off a windshield. But targeted

70

affirmations—ones that speak directly to your core wounds—can gradually rewire your default thoughts [32].

Here are morning affirmations crafted for each schema:

For Abandonment Schema:

- "I am whole and complete on my own"
- "People who truly care about me want to stay"
- "I can handle life's natural comings and goings"

For Mistrust Schema:

- "I can distinguish between actual threats and old fears"
- "There are trustworthy people in the world, and I can find them"
- "I am learning to trust wisely, not blindly"

For Emotional Deprivation:

- "My emotional needs are valid and important"
- "I am learning to recognize and receive care"
- "There are people who want to understand me"

For Defectiveness Schema:

- "I am worthy of love exactly as I am"
- "My imperfections make me human, not unlovable"
- "I deserve kindness, especially from myself"

For Social Isolation:

- "I belong here as much as anyone"

- "My unique perspective adds value"
- "Connection is possible when I show up authentically"

For Dependence Schema:

- "I am more capable than my fears suggest"
- "I can handle challenges one step at a time"
- "Asking for help is wisdom, not weakness"

For Vulnerability Schema:

- "I am safer than my nervous system believes"
- "I can cope with uncertainty"
- "Most of what I fear never happens"

For Enmeshment Schema:

- "I am a separate person with my own valid needs"
- "Healthy boundaries create healthier relationships"
- "I can care about others and still be myself"

For Failure Schema:

- "I am competent and continue learning"
- "Mistakes are information, not verdicts"
- "My worth isn't determined by achievements"

For Entitlement Schema:

- "I am special AND so is everyone else"
- "Rules help create safety for everyone, including me"

- "I can meet my needs while respecting others"

For Insufficient Self-Control:

- "I am building discipline with patience"
- "Small consistent actions create big changes"
- "I can pause between impulse and action"

For Subjugation Schema:

- "My needs matter as much as anyone's"
- "I can be kind AND have boundaries"
- "Saying no to others means saying yes to myself"

For Self-Sacrifice Schema:

- "Taking care of myself helps me care for others"
- "I deserve the same compassion I give"
- "Balance serves everyone better than burnout"

For Approval-Seeking Schema:

- "I approve of myself, and that's enough"
- "Not everyone needs to like me"
- "My worth comes from within, not from others' opinions"

For Negativity Schema:

- "Good things happen too, and I can notice them"
- "Today might surprise me with joy"
- "I can hold both caution and hope"

For Emotional Inhibition:

- "My emotions are safe to feel and express"
- "Vulnerability is courage, not weakness"
- "I can stay in control while still feeling"

For Unrelenting Standards:

- "Good enough is genuinely good enough"
- "I am human, not a machine"
- "Rest is productive too"

For Punitiveness Schema:

- "Everyone deserves compassion, including me"
- "Mistakes are chances to learn, not reasons for punishment"
- "I can be accountable without being harsh"

Making Affirmations Work

Simply reciting words won't override decades of neural programming. Here's how to make affirmations effective:

1. **Say them looking at yourself** in the mirror—this activates self-recognition areas of the brain

2. **Place your hand on your heart** while speaking—this activates the soothing system

3. **Start with "I am learning to..."** if the full affirmation feels too unbelievable

4. **Record them in your own voice** and listen during morning routines

5. **Write them down** after saying them—this engages multiple brain pathways

Intention Setting for the Day

After affirmations, set one schema-healing intention for the day. This isn't a to-do list item but a way of being:

- "Today I'll notice when I'm assuming abandonment"

- "Today I'll practice believing I'm good enough"

- "Today I'll honor one of my own needs"

- "Today I'll celebrate one imperfect action"

Write this intention on a sticky note where you'll see it repeatedly—bathroom mirror, computer screen, car dashboard.

Case Example 1: Rachel's Morning Revolution

Rachel's subjugation schema had her checking work emails before getting out of bed, immediately prioritizing everyone else's needs. Her new morning routine:

1. **Phone stays outside bedroom** (radical but effective)

2. **First thought replacement**: Instead of "What does everyone need?" she asks "What do I need?"

3. **Mirror affirmation**: "My needs matter. I can help others AND honor myself"

4. **Intention setting**: Each day, one small way to honor her own needs

5. **5-minute meditation**: Using an app with a self-compassion focus

"The first week felt selfish and wrong," Rachel shared. "But by week three, I noticed I had more energy for others because I wasn't starting the day already depleted. My schema still whispers, but it doesn't get the microphone first thing anymore" [33].

5-Minute Guided Meditations

Meditation helps you observe schemas without being controlled by them. These brief morning meditations target schema healing:

Basic Schema Awareness Meditation:

1. Sit comfortably, close your eyes

2. Take three deep breaths

3. Notice what thoughts are present

4. Label schema thoughts: "Ah, abandonment speaking" or "Hello, perfectionism"

5. Return to breath without judging

6. End with one compassionate statement to yourself

Inner Child Morning Check-In:

1. Breathe deeply, hand on heart

2. Visualize your inner child

3. Ask: "How are you this morning?"

4. Listen without trying to fix

5. Offer one comforting message

6. Promise to check in later

Future Self Meditation:

1. Relax and breathe naturally

2. Visualize yourself one year from now

3. See yourself with healed schemas

4. Notice how you move, speak, feel

5. Ask future self for one piece of wisdom

6. Thank them and return to present

Throughout the Day

Schemas don't just attack in the morning—they're opportunistic, waiting for moments of stress, uncertainty, or trigger to activate. Having tools ready throughout the day helps you respond rather than react.

The STOP Technique

When you notice schema activation, STOP:

S - Stop: Pause whatever you're doing. Just freeze for a moment.

T - Take a breath: One deep breath activates the parasympathetic nervous system, moving you out of fight-or-flight.

O - Observe:

- What triggered this?

- Which schema is active?

- What is my schema telling me?

- What am I feeling in my body?

P - Proceed with choice:

- How would I respond without this schema?

- What would self-compassion do here?

- What small action aligns with my healing?

Case Example 2: Mark's STOP Success

Mark's entitlement schema activated when a car cut him off in traffic. His usual response was rage, honking, and aggressive driving to "teach them a lesson." Using STOP:

S: He gripped the wheel but didn't accelerate **T**: Deep breath through the nose **O**: "Entitlement schema says 'How dare they disrespect me!' Body is tense, jaw clenched" **P**: "Without this schema, it's just traffic. I'll stay in my lane, play calming music"

"First time I tried STOP, I felt like a pushover," Mark admitted. "But I arrived at work calm instead of furious. That was worth more than 'winning' against a stranger I'll never see again" [34].

Schema Alerts Recognizing Activation

Create a personal alert system for schema activation. Common early warning signs:

Body Alerts:

- Chest tightening (abandonment)

- Jaw clenching (punitiveness)

- Stomach dropping (failure)

- Shoulders rising (vulnerability)

- Feeling small (defectiveness)

Thought Alerts (key phrases that signal activation):

- "Here we go again..." (pessimism)
- "I knew this would happen..." (mistrust)
- "I should have..." (unrelenting standards)
- "Why do I even try..." (failure)
- "No one understands..." (emotional deprivation)

Behavioral Alerts:

- Checking phone obsessively (abandonment)
- Redoing completed work (perfectionism)
- Saying yes when you mean no (subjugation)
- Withdrawing suddenly (defectiveness)
- Testing people (mistrust)

When you notice an alert, that's your cue to use STOP or another coping strategy.

In-the-Moment Coping Cards

Create pocket-sized cards for schema emergencies. Each card has:

- The schema name
- A grounding statement
- One quick action
- A reminder of reality

Example cards:

Abandonment Emergency Card: "This feeling is familiar, not factual. Breathe. Text a stable friend. People leave AND people stay. You survived before, you'll survive now."

Perfectionism Emergency Card: "Excellence isn't required right now. Breathe. Do 'good enough.' Mistakes don't equal unworthiness. Progress, not perfection."

Subjugation Emergency Card: "Your needs matter too. Breathe. State one need clearly. Disappointing others won't kill you. You can be kind AND have boundaries."

Evening Reflection

Evenings offer a chance to consolidate learning and celebrate progress. This isn't about judging your day but about noticing patterns with curiosity and compassion.

The Schema Journal Format

Dedicate 10 minutes each evening to schema reflection:

Date: _____

Schema Activations Today: Which schemas showed up? _____ What triggered them? _____

Old Pattern Responses: How did I initially react?

_____

New Responses I Tried: What did I do differently?

_____

What I Learned: About my triggers:

_____ About my capacity: _____

Tomorrow's Opportunity: One situation where I can practice: _____

Gratitude for Growth: One small way I'm different than before: _____

Celebrating Small Wins

Schemas thrive on criticism and minimize progress. Counter this by deliberately celebrating:

Daily Win Categories:

- **Awareness wins**: "I noticed my schema in real-time"
- **Pause wins**: "I stopped before reacting automatically"
- **Choice wins**: "I tried something different, even if small"
- **Recovery wins**: "I got hijacked but came back faster"
- **Courage wins**: "I felt the fear and acted anyway"

Create a "Win Jar"—write each win on a slip of paper and add to a jar. On hard days, read past wins to remember your progress.

Case Example 3: Sofia's Evening Revolution

Sofia's failure schema had her reviewing each day for evidence of incompetence. Her new evening practice:

1. **Timer for 10 minutes** (no endless rumination)
2. **Start with wins**, however tiny
3. **Note schema stories** versus actual facts
4. **Write tomorrow's experiment**

5. **End with self-compassion statement**

"My journal showed me patterns I'd never noticed," Sofia reflected. "Like how my failure schema activated most on Mondays and before meetings. Now I prepare extra self-care for those times. Also, reading back, I see I haven't been fired, demoted, or even criticized—my schema was lying" [35].

Planning Tomorrow's Practice

End each evening by planning one schema-healing practice for tomorrow:

- "I'll wait 5 minutes before saying yes to requests"

- "I'll share one opinion in the team meeting"

- "I'll leave work on time without apologizing"

- "I'll compliment myself for one thing"

Keep it specific, small, and doable. Success builds on success.

Chapter Tools

Tear-Out Affirmation Cards

Create personal affirmation cards for different situations:

Morning Card: Core affirmation for daily use **Pocket Card**: Quick reminder for challenging moments **Mirror Card**: Taped where you'll see it **Phone Card**: Photo on phone for discrete viewing **Crisis Card**: For highest activation moments

Decorate them, laminate them, make them yours. The act of creating them is healing in itself.

Pocket Coping Cards

Beyond schema-specific cards, create situation cards:

Before Difficult Conversations: "I can speak my truth calmly. Their reaction is about them. I deserve respect. Breathe between sentences."

When Triggered at Work: "This job doesn't define me. One task at a time. Perfect isn't the goal. I belong here."

In Social Situations: "I don't need to perform. Being myself is enough. Not everyone has to like me. I can leave when ready."

Schema Journal Template

Weekly Review Page:

This Week's Primary Schema:

_____

Times It Activated:

_____

Old Patterns:

_____

New Responses Tried:

_____

Success Rate: ____/10

Key Learning:

_____

Next Week's Focus:

_____

Self-Compassion Note:

_____

Living the Daily Practice

Schema healing isn't a dramatic transformation—it's a daily practice of small, conscious choices. Each morning affirmation slightly weakens your schema's morning assault. Each STOP technique creates space between trigger and response. Each evening reflection builds self-awareness. Each celebrated win rewires your brain toward self-compassion.

Some days, you'll forget everything and fall into old patterns. That's not failure—it's being human. The difference now is you have tools to find your way back. You're not trying to never have schema activations; you're building a life where schemas don't run the show.

Your daily practices are like water on stone—individually, each drop seems insignificant, but over time, they reshape the hardest surfaces. Be patient with yourself. You're rewriting decades of programming, one morning, one breath, one choice at a time.

Key Takeaways

- **Morning practices** set neural pathways for the entire day

- **Schema-specific affirmations** work better than generic positive thinking

- **Daily intentions** focus on ways of being, not just doing

- **The STOP technique** creates choice points during schema activation

- **Body, thought, and behavior alerts** signal when schemas are taking over

- **Coping cards** provide immediate support during difficult moments

- **Evening journaling** consolidates learning and reveals patterns

- **Celebrating small wins** counters schemas' tendency to minimize progress

- **Consistency matters more** than perfection in daily practices

- **Tools work best** when personalized to your specific schemas and life

You now have a full toolkit for daily schema work—morning practices to start strong, throughout-the-day techniques for challenges, and evening reflections for growth. But healing happens best in connection with others. In our next chapter, we'll explore how schemas play out in relationships and how to create healthier patterns with the people who matter most.

Chapter 7: Relationships and Schemas

Two magnets sit on opposite ends of a table. Slowly push them together and watch what happens—they'll either snap together with surprising force or repel each other, spinning away. This is exactly how schemas operate in relationships. Sarah, with her abandonment schema, found herself drawn to James, whose emotional unavailability triggered every abandonment fear she had. Meanwhile, she felt "no chemistry" with stable, consistent Mark who texted when he said he would and showed up reliably. "There's just no spark," she told friends, unable to recognize that her schema interpreted safety as boredom and chaos as connection. Our schemas don't just affect how we behave in relationships—they determine who we're attracted to in the first place.

Schema Chemistry Why We Attract Certain People

Your schemas act like relationship magnets, drawing you toward people who feel familiar—not necessarily people who are good for you. This "schema chemistry" explains why you might find yourself in the same painful relationship dynamics with different people, wondering how you keep ending up here.

The Familiarity Trap: Your brain equates familiar with safe, even when familiar means painful. If you grew up walking on eggshells around an unpredictable parent, a partner's mood swings might feel like home. If love meant earning approval through achievement, you'll be drawn to partners whose affection feels conditional.

Common Schema Attractions:

- **Abandonment attracts**: Emotionally unavailable partners, people who give mixed signals, those with one foot out the door

- **Defectiveness attracts**: Critical partners, those who need "fixing," people who confirm your unworthiness

- **Subjugation attracts**: Dominant personalities, people with strong opinions, those who need caretaking

- **Emotional deprivation attracts**: Partners who struggle with intimacy, emotionally shut down types

- **Mistrust attracts**: Secretive people, those with poor boundaries, partners who trigger detective mode

- **Failure attracts**: Highly critical people, perfectionists, those who highlight your inadequacies

- **Unrelenting standards attracts**: Other perfectionists, or opposites who you can "improve"

Case Example 1: Maria's Pattern Recognition

Maria, 34, sat in therapy listing her ex-boyfriends: "Jake was a workaholic who canceled half our dates. Ryan was still hung up on his ex. Alex would disappear for days without explanation. Tom was married—I didn't know at first." Her therapist asked what they had in common. Maria laughed bitterly: "They were all emotionally unavailable jerks?"

"Or," her therapist suggested gently, "they all activated your abandonment schema. The 'chemistry' you felt was your schema recognizing a familiar pattern."

Maria's mind was blown. She realized she'd friend-zoned every emotionally available man she'd met. "Dave from work asked me out last year. He's kind, stable, texts back quickly. I told everyone he was 'too nice' and I wasn't attracted. But maybe... maybe my schema just didn't recognize him?" [36]

Breaking Old Patterns

Breaking relationship patterns requires conscious effort across all relationship types. Your schemas don't limit themselves to romance—they show up with family, friends, and colleagues too.

In Romantic Relationships

Step 1: Recognize Your Pattern Map out your relationship history. Look for:

- Similar types you're attracted to
- Repeated conflicts across relationships
- How relationships typically end
- Your role in the pattern

Step 2: Identify Schema Triggers

- What makes you feel instantly attracted?
- What behaviors make you anxious?
- When do you feel most secure/insecure?

Step 3: Date Against Type (Consciously)

- If you usually date extroverts, try an introvert
- If you chase unavailable people, date someone enthusiastic about you

- If you pick projects to fix, choose someone stable

Step 4: Tolerate "Boring" (It's Not Really Boring) Schema chemistry feels exciting because it activates your nervous system. Healthy relationships might feel "flat" at first because they're not triggering fight-or-flight. Give it time.

Step 5: Communicate Your Schema Work "I'm working on some old patterns from my past. Sometimes I might react strongly to things that seem small. I'm learning to separate past from present."

Case Example 2: Tom's Romantic Revolution

Tom's subjugation schema had him in relationships where he was always the giver. His partners made the plans, chose the restaurants, decided the relationship pace. When he started dating Emma, he practiced small assertions:

- Week 1: "Actually, I'd prefer Italian over sushi tonight"

- Week 3: "I need some alone time this weekend to recharge"

- Week 6: "I'm not comfortable moving in together yet"

"Each time I expected Emma to leave," Tom shared. "Instead, she said things like 'Thanks for telling me what you need.' My schema kept insisting she'd get angry, but reality kept proving it wrong" [37].

With Family Members

Family relationships are schema ground zero—where patterns began and where they're most entrenched. Change here is possible but requires adjusted expectations.

The Family Schema Dance: Families operate like choreographed dances. Everyone knows their steps. When you change your moves, expect confusion and resistance.

Strategies for Family Pattern Breaking:

1. **Start Small**: Don't announce you're breaking patterns. Just start responding differently.

2. **Use the Broken Record Technique**: Calmly repeat your boundary without justifying

   - "I won't be discussing my weight"

   - "I said I won't be discussing my weight"

   - "Let's talk about something else. I won't discuss my weight"

3. **Have Exit Strategies**: "I'll need to leave if this continues" (and follow through)

4. **Find Your Allies**: Usually one family member is ready for healthier dynamics

5. **Grieve the Fantasy**: Accept they might never be the family you needed

In Friendships

Friendships often recreate family dynamics. The "best friend" who criticizes everything might echo a critical parent. The friend who always needs rescuing might trigger your self-sacrifice schema.

Friendship Pattern Breakers:

- **Notice Role Assignments**: Are you always the listener? The organizer? The one who apologizes?

- **Test New Behaviors**: If you're always the helper, ask for help. If you're the entertainment, let others lead conversation.

- **Diversify Your Friend Group**: Different friends can meet different needs

- **Quality Over Quantity**: One healthy friendship beats five schema-triggering ones

At Work

Work relationships activate schemas powerfully because they involve hierarchy, evaluation, and financial security—all schema triggers.

Common Work Schema Patterns:

- Subjugation: Never disagreeing with boss, overworking

- Failure: Avoiding visibility, declining promotions

- Unrelenting Standards: Perfectionism that slows productivity

- Entitlement: Conflict with authority, rule-breaking

Breaking Work Patterns:

1. Identify your work schema triggers (criticism, authority, deadlines)

2. Practice one small change weekly

3. Find a work mentor who models healthy patterns

4. Separate current boss from past authority figures

Case Example 3: Ana's Workplace Transformation

Ana's defectiveness schema made her interpret every piece of feedback as proof she didn't belong. When her manager said, "Great presentation, next time maybe include more visuals," Ana heard, "You're incompetent and we're building a case to fire you."

Her schema work included:

- Writing down exact words said versus her interpretation

- Asking clarifying questions: "Overall, how did you feel about the presentation?"

- Noticing colleagues receiving similar feedback without catastrophe

- Practicing self-compassion: "Feedback helps me grow, it's not an attack"

After six months, Ana reported: "I actually asked my boss for feedback yesterday. Old me would never believe it. When she gave suggestions, I took notes instead of planning my resignation" [38].

Healthy Communication Scripts

Schemas make communication feel dangerous. Here are scripts that honor your needs while respecting others:

Expressing Needs Despite Vulnerability Schemas

When vulnerability schemas make expressing needs feel dangerous:

Instead of: Suffering in silence or exploding later **Try**: "I have something I need to share, and I'm feeling vulnerable about it. Could we talk when you have 10 minutes?"

Script for Sharing Needs: "I've noticed I need [specific thing]. I know this might be different from what we usually do. Can we figure out how to make this work for both of us?"

If They React Poorly: "I can see this surprised you. I'm still learning to express my needs. Can we revisit this when we've both had time to think?"

Setting Boundaries Despite Subjugation Schemas

When subjugation schemas make boundaries feel selfish:

The Boundary Sandwich:

1. Acknowledge: "I understand this is important to you..."

2. Boundary: "...and I'm not able to do that..."

3. Alternative: "...but I could do [alternative] instead."

Examples:

- "I understand you need help moving this weekend, and I'm not available Saturday, but I could help you pack boxes Friday evening."

- "I hear that you're upset, and I'm not comfortable being yelled at, but I'm happy to discuss this when we're both calmer."

For Persistent Pushers: "I've thought about it, and my answer is still no. I hope you can respect that."

Asking for Help Despite Self-Reliance Schemas

When self-reliance schemas make asking for help feel weak:

Start with Acknowledgment: "This is hard for me to ask..." "I usually handle things myself, but..." "I'm practicing asking for support, so..."

Make Specific Requests: Instead of: "I'm drowning, I need help with everything" Try: "Could you pick up groceries this week? I'm overwhelmed with the project deadline."

Scripts for Different Situations:

Emotional Support: "I'm going through something difficult. Could you listen for 10 minutes? I don't need solutions, just a caring ear."

Practical Help: "I'm learning to ask for help when needed. Would you be willing to [specific task]? If not, no worries."

Professional Assistance: "I've always prided myself on figuring things out alone, but I think I need guidance with this. Could we schedule time to discuss?"

Chapter Exercise "Relationship Schema Map"

Create a visual map of how your schemas show up in relationships:

Part 1: Relationship Inventory

List significant relationships (past and present):

1. _____ Type: _____

2. _____ Type: _____

3. _____ Type: _____

4. _____ Type: _____

5. _____ Type: _____

Part 2: Pattern Recognition

For each relationship, note:

- Which of your schemas activated most?
- Which of their likely schemas interacted with yours?
- Repeated conflicts or dynamics?
- How did it end (or current status)?

Part 3: Schema Chemistry Analysis

Draw lines connecting similar patterns across relationships. Notice:

- Do you attract similar types?
- Do similar conflicts repeat?
- What role do you typically play?

Part 4: Healthy Relationship Vision

Describe a relationship without schema interference:

- How would you feel? _____
- How would you communicate? _____
- What would be different? _____
- What might challenge your schemas? _____

Part 5: Action Steps

Three specific things to try in current relationships:

1. In romantic/potential romantic: _____
2. With family: _____

3. With friends: _____

Part 6: Support Network

Identify people who support your schema healing:

- Who models healthy patterns? _____
- Who can you practice with? _____
- Who celebrates your growth? _____

Moving Forward in Connection

Relationships are where schemas learned their tricks, and relationships are where they heal. Every interaction offers a chance to respond from your adult self rather than your wounded child. Some people will celebrate your growth. Others might resist, preferring the old, predictable you. This sorting process—while painful—leads to more authentic connections.

You're not trying to have perfect relationships or eliminate all conflict. You're learning to recognize when schemas hijack interactions and choosing responses aligned with who you're becoming. Each healthy interaction rewrites your relational blueprint, proving your schemas wrong one connection at a time.

Key Takeaways

- **Schema chemistry** creates attraction to familiar (not healthy) relationship dynamics
- **We attract partners** who activate our deepest schemas, mistaking intensity for love
- **Breaking patterns requires** conscious choice to date/befriend "against type"

- **Family patterns** are most entrenched but small changes create ripple effects

- **Work relationships** activate schemas through hierarchy and evaluation

- **Healthy communication** requires scripts that overcome schema fears

- **Boundary setting** gets easier with practice and pre-planned phrases

- **Asking for help** challenges self-reliance schemas but deepens connections

- **Relationship mapping** reveals patterns across all relationship types

- **Growth in relationships** means some people celebrate while others resist

As you practice new relationship patterns, expect setbacks. Your schemas have been protecting you in relationships for years—they won't retire without a fight. In our next chapter, we'll explore how to handle these inevitable setbacks with compassion rather than criticism.

Chapter 8: Setbacks and Self-Compassion

The email arrived at 3 PM on a Thursday. "We've decided to go with another candidate." Rachel stared at the screen, feeling her chest tighten in a familiar way. She'd worked so hard on her failure schema, done months of exercises, practiced self-compassion. Yet here it was, flooding back full force: "Of course you didn't get it. You're not good enough. You'll never be good enough. All that schema work was just pretending." By 3:15, Rachel had canceled her evening plans, decided to skip her friend's birthday party that weekend, and was mentally composing her resignation from her current job because "what's the point?" Six months of progress felt erased in six minutes. But then, something different happened. Rachel noticed herself spiraling. She put her hand on her heart and whispered, "This is a setback, not a setup. I know what to do." The schema was loud, but for the first time, it wasn't the only voice in the room.

Why Setbacks Happen

Setbacks aren't just normal in schema work—they're inevitable. Understanding why helps you prepare for and navigate them with less self-attack.

The Brain's Preference for Familiar

Your brain is remarkably efficient, and efficiency loves the familiar. Think about driving a route you've taken hundreds of times—you arrive without remembering most of the journey. Your brain automated the process. Schemas work the same way. They're your brain's automated responses to certain triggers, carved deep through years of repetition [39].

When you start practicing new responses, you're essentially asking your brain to take the scenic route instead of the highway it's used to. This requires:

- More conscious effort
- More energy expenditure
- More attention and focus
- More uncertainty tolerance

Under stress, your brain defaults to its most efficient option: the old schema highway. This isn't weakness or failure—it's neurology.

The Groove Metaphor: Imagine water flowing down a hillside. Over time, it carves a groove. Even if you dig a new path for the water, during heavy rain, it tends to flow back into the deeper, original groove. Your schemas are deep grooves. New patterns are shallow scratches. Time and repetition deepen new grooves, but heavy emotional rain still finds old paths.

Stress and Schema Reactivation

Stress is schemas' best friend. When your resources are depleted, schemas stage comebacks like retired boxers returning for one more fight. Common stress triggers that reactivate schemas:

Physical Depletion:

- Lack of sleep
- Hunger or poor nutrition
- Illness or pain

- Hormonal changes
- Substance use

Emotional Overload:

- Grief or loss
- Major life transitions
- Relationship conflicts
- Work pressure
- Financial stress

Anniversary Reactions:

- Time of year when trauma occurred
- Ages when schemas formed
- Holidays or significant dates
- Sensory triggers (smells, sounds)

Case Example 1: Marcus's Perfect Storm

Marcus had made tremendous progress with his unrelenting standards schema. He was submitting "good enough" work, taking breaks, even making intentional mistakes. Then came the perfect storm:

- His father visited (critic trigger)
- Annual performance review approached (evaluation trigger)
- He got flu (physical depletion)
- His girlfriend mentioned marriage (vulnerability trigger)

"It was like I'd never done any work at all," Marcus reported. "I stayed until midnight 'perfecting' a routine report. I redid my apartment cleaning three times before Dad arrived. I wrote and rewrote a simple email seventeen times. My schema came back like it had been doing pushups, stronger than ever" [40].

It's Not Failure, It's Data

Reframe setbacks as data collection rather than failure. Each setback provides information about:

- Which situations remain triggering
- What stress levels overwhelm new patterns
- Where more support is needed
- Which tools work during crisis
- How quickly you can recover

The Scientist Mindset Returns: "Interesting. My abandonment schema reactivated when my friend canceled lunch during my work deadline stress. Data point: Combined social and work stress still overwhelms my new patterns. Hypothesis: I need stronger coping strategies for multi-domain stress."

The Self-Compassion Toolkit

Self-compassion isn't soft or weak—it's the strongest response to setbacks. Research shows self-compassion leads to more behavior change than self-criticism, not less [41].

Kristen Neff's Three Components Simplified

Dr. Kristen Neff identified three components of self-compassion. Here's how to apply them to schema setbacks:

1. Mindfulness (Noticing without drowning)

- Observe your pain without minimizing or exaggerating
- "I'm noticing my failure schema is really active right now"
- "I feel ashamed and want to hide"
- Not: "I'm the worst" or "This is nothing"

2. Common Humanity (You're not alone)

- Everyone has setbacks
- Schemas affect millions of people
- Your struggle is part of human experience
- "Other people working on schemas have setbacks too"

3. Self-Kindness (Treat yourself like a good friend)

- What would you say to a friend in this situation?
- Offer yourself the same understanding
- "This is a hard moment. What do I need right now?"

Self-Compassion Phrases for Each Schema

Memorize one or two phrases for your primary schemas. During setbacks, these become life rafts:

Abandonment: "Being left hurts, and I'm still here for myself. This feeling will pass."

Mistrust: "It's hard to trust after being hurt. I'm learning to trust wisely."

Emotional Deprivation: "I deserve care and understanding, starting with my own."

Defectiveness: "I am whole and worthy, even in difficult moments."

Social Isolation: "Feeling different is painful. I belong in this world."

Dependence: "Asking for help shows wisdom. I'm more capable than I feel."

Vulnerability: "Fear is trying to protect me. I'm safer than my schema believes."

Enmeshment: "I can care about others and still be separate."

Failure: "Mistakes are human. They don't define my worth."

Entitlement: "I matter, and so does everyone else."

Insufficient Self-Control: "I'm building new patterns. Progress isn't always linear."

Subjugation: "My needs matter. I'm learning to honor them."

Self-Sacrifice: "Caring for myself allows me to care for others."

Approval-Seeking: "I approve of myself, especially when struggling."

Negativity: "Hard things happen. Good things happen too."

Emotional Inhibition: "Feelings are safe to have, even difficult ones."

Unrelenting Standards: "I'm human, not a machine. Good enough is enough."

Punitiveness: "Everyone deserves compassion during setbacks, including me."

The "Best Friend" Technique

When self-compassion feels impossible, use this powerful redirect:

1. **Imagine your best friend** came to you with exactly your situation
2. **What would you say** to them?
3. **What would you absolutely NOT say** to them?
4. **What comfort would you offer**?
5. **Now give that to yourself**

Case Example 2: Elena's Best Friend Breakthrough

Elena's abandonment schema reactivated when her boyfriend went on a business trip without much contact. She found herself checking his social media obsessively, convinced he was cheating.

"I was calling myself 'pathetic' and 'crazy,'" Elena shared. "Then I pictured my best friend Sarah in this exact situation. Would I call Sarah pathetic? Never. I'd say, 'Your feelings make sense given your history. Let's find ways to soothe this anxiety that don't involve detective work.' So I became my own best friend that night" [42].

Getting Back on Track

Recovery from setbacks follows predictable patterns. Having a plan speeds the process.

The 24-Hour Rule

Give yourself 24 hours to feel the setback fully before taking action:

Hour 0-6: Feel the feelings. Cry, journal, talk to someone safe. Don't make big decisions.

Hour 6-12: Basic self-care. Shower, eat, gentle movement. Still no big decisions.

Hour 12-18: Review your tools. What's helped before? Small self-compassion gestures.

Hour 18-24: Make one small plan. What's the tiniest step back toward your growth?

After 24 Hours: Implement your small plan. Build from there.

Micro-Restarts

You don't need a dramatic comeback. Micro-restarts get you moving without overwhelming your depleted system:

- Read one page of your schema journal
- Say one affirmation
- Text one supportive friend
- Do one breathing exercise
- Write one self-compassion phrase
- Practice one boundary for five minutes

Each micro-restart is a vote for recovery over surrender.

Progress Tracking That Motivates

During setbacks, your schema will insist you've made no progress. Combat this with evidence:

The Progress Photo Album (Metaphorical or Literal):

- Keep screenshots of breakthrough moments
- Save supportive texts from friends
- Document small wins in a special notebook
- Create a "Evidence I'm Growing" file

The Setback Timeline: Track your setback patterns over time:

- How long do they typically last?
- Are they getting shorter?
- Is recovery getting faster?
- Are triggers becoming more specific?

Case Example 3: David's Data-Driven Recovery

David's subjugation schema roared back during family holidays. He found himself saying yes to everything, exhausting himself with people-pleasing. But he'd been tracking:

"First holiday after starting schema work: 2-week recovery
Second holiday: 10-day recovery
Third holiday: 5-day recovery Fourth holiday: 2-day recovery

Last holiday, I noticed the pattern starting and used my tools immediately. I still had setback moments, but I could say,

'Based on data, I'll feel more myself in 48 hours.' And I did" [43].

Chapter Exercise "My Compassion Plan"

Create your personalized setback recovery plan while you're feeling strong:

Part 1: Early Warning Signs My schema reactivation warning signs:

- Physical: _____
- Emotional: _____
- Thoughts: _____
- Behaviors: _____

Part 2: My Compassion Phrases Write 3 phrases that soothe your specific schema:

1. _____
2. _____
3. _____

Part 3: My Support Network People I can reach out to during setbacks:

- For listening: _____
- For distraction: _____
- For gentle accountability: _____

Part 4: My Micro-Restart Menu 5 tiny actions I can take when overwhelmed:

1. _____

2. _____

3. _____

4. _____

5. _____

Part 5: My Progress Evidence Where I keep proof of growth:

- Physical location: _____

- Digital location: _____

- One progress moment to remember: _____

Part 6: My 24-Hour Plan Hour 0-6, I will:
_____ Hour 6-12, I will:
_____ Hour 12-18, I will:
_____ Hour 18-24, I will:
_____

Part 7: My Comeback Statement One sentence to read during setbacks:

_____

_____

The Spiral Path Forward

Schema healing isn't a straight line from wounded to well. It's a spiral path where you revisit familiar territory from higher ground. That rejection that once devastated you for months might now sting for days. The criticism that once confirmed your worthlessness might now prompt curiosity about the critic's bad day.

Setbacks aren't evidence that schema work doesn't work— they're evidence that you're human, living a full life with all its triggers and challenges. Each setback handled with compassion rather than criticism rewires your brain a little more. You're not just healing schemas; you're learning to be kind to yourself when life gets hard. That's a skill worth more than never having setbacks at all.

Key Takeaways

- **Setbacks are inevitable** because brains prefer familiar neural pathways

- **Stress reactivates schemas** by depleting the resources needed for new patterns

- **Physical depletion** makes you vulnerable to schema reactivation

- **Setbacks provide data** about triggers, needs, and recovery patterns

- **Self-compassion has three parts**: mindfulness, common humanity, and self-kindness

- **Schema-specific phrases** help during crisis when generating compassion feels hard

- **The "best friend" technique** bypasses self-criticism by redirecting care

- **The 24-hour rule** prevents impulsive decisions during peak activation

- **Micro-restarts** get you moving without overwhelming depleted resources

- **Progress tracking** combats schema lies about "no improvement"

- **Recovery gets faster** with practice, even if setbacks still occur

You've learned to work with your schemas, test new beliefs, practice daily tools, navigate relationships, and now handle setbacks with compassion. Sometimes, despite your best efforts, you might need professional support. In our final chapter, we'll explore when and how to seek help, and how therapy can amplify your self-help journey.

Chapter 9: When to Seek Professional Help

Dr. Sarah Chen had been a therapist for fifteen years, but she still remembered her first schema therapy session as a client. "I'd read all the self-help books," she told her supervisor during training. "I'd done the exercises, kept the journals, practiced the techniques. But sitting across from someone trained to hold space for my schemas—it was like the difference between reading about swimming and actually getting in the water with an instructor." Now, as clients asked her the same question she'd once wondered— "When do I need professional help?"—she'd share her truth: "Self-help can take you far. Sometimes, though, you need a skilled guide for the deeper waters. There's no shame in that. There's wisdom."

Signs You Might Benefit from Therapy

Seeking professional help isn't a sign of failure—it's a sign of commitment to your healing. Here are indicators that therapy might be your next step:

Self-Assessment Checklist

Check any that apply to your current experience:

Intensity Indicators: ☐ Schemas interfere with daily functioning (work, relationships, self-care) ☐ Emotional pain feels unbearable or constant ☐ You're having thoughts of self-harm or suicide ☐ Anxiety or depression alongside schemas feels unmanageable ☐ Physical symptoms (panic attacks, insomnia, appetite changes) persist

Duration Indicators: ☐ You've been working alone for 6+ months with minimal progress ☐ Setbacks last longer than a few days ☐ The same patterns repeat despite your efforts ☐ You feel stuck in the same schema stories

Complexity Indicators: ☐ Multiple schemas activate simultaneously ☐ Trauma memories surface during schema work ☐ You dissociate or "check out" when triggered ☐ Childhood memories are largely blank or confusing ☐ You suspect deeper issues beneath schemas

Relationship Indicators: ☐ Schemas damage important relationships repeatedly ☐ You can't maintain any close relationships ☐ People express concern about your patterns ☐ Isolation feels safer than connection

Coping Indicators: ☐ You're using substances to manage schema pain ☐ Self-harm behaviors provide relief ☐ Eating, spending, or sex used to numb feelings ☐ Can't self-soothe during activation

Support Indicators: ☐ Limited social support system ☐ Family of origin still heavily triggers schemas ☐ Current life stress exceeds coping capacity ☐ Need someone to be accountable to

If you checked 3+ boxes, therapy could significantly help. If you checked any in the "Intensity" category, especially self-harm thoughts, please reach out for professional support today.

When Self-Help Isn't Enough

Self-help works beautifully for many people, but some situations need professional support:

Complex Trauma: If schemas stem from severe abuse, neglect, or repeated trauma, professional help provides necessary safety and expertise.

Blind Spots: We can't see our own patterns fully. A therapist offers an outside perspective on dynamics you might miss.

Skill Building: Some techniques (like imagery rescripting or chair work) work best with professional guidance initially.

Accountability: Weekly appointments create structure and momentum that self-help sometimes lacks.

Relationship Laboratory: The therapeutic relationship itself becomes a place to practice new patterns safely.

Case Example 1: Jennifer's Recognition

Jennifer worked on her abandonment schema for eight months using self-help books. She made progress—less texting anxiety, better boundary setting. But certain triggers still sent her into multi-day spirals.

"I realized I needed help when my boyfriend went on a guys' weekend and I spent 48 hours convinced he was leaving me," Jennifer shared. "I'd used every tool I knew, but I was still checking his location, calling friends to analyze his texts, and preparing for breakup. That's when I knew I needed professional support" [44].

Finding a Schema Therapist

Not all therapists are trained in schema therapy. Here's how to find someone who can specifically help with schema work:

What to Look For

Essential Qualifications:

- Licensed mental health professional (psychologist, counselor, social worker)
- Specific training in schema therapy
- Experience with your presenting concerns
- Good therapeutic alliance (you feel comfortable)

Ideal Additions:

- Certified by International Society of Schema Therapy (ISST)
- Regular consultation/supervision in schema therapy
- Additional trauma training (if relevant)
- Experience with your specific schemas

Green Flags:

- Explains schema therapy clearly
- Balances warmth with boundaries
- Shows genuine empathy
- Discusses treatment timeline
- Collaborative approach

Red Flags:

- Promises quick fixes
- Seems judgmental about schemas
- No specific schema therapy training
- Inflexible approach

- Poor boundaries (too distant or too friendly)

Questions to Ask

During consultation calls or first sessions, ask:

About Training: "What specific training do you have in schema therapy?" "How long have you been practicing schema therapy?" "Do you receive ongoing consultation?"

About Approach: "How do you typically work with [your specific schemas]?" "What's your treatment approach for schema therapy?" "How do you integrate other modalities?"

About Practicalities: "What's the typical frequency of sessions?" "How long does schema therapy usually take?" "What's your fee, and do you offer sliding scale?" "Do you assign homework between sessions?"

About Fit: "What's your experience with clients like me?" "How do you handle setbacks in therapy?" "What's your approach to the therapeutic relationship?"

Online Directories and Resources

International Society of Schema Therapy (ISST)

- Website: isst.com

- Features: Find a therapist directory by location

- Verification: Lists certified schema therapists

Psychology Today

- Website: psychologytoday.com

- Features: Searchable by location, insurance, specialty

- Note: Filter for "schema therapy" in specialties

Your Insurance Provider

- Call for in-network providers
- Ask specifically about schema therapy coverage
- Request names to research further

Local Training Institutes

- Universities with clinical psychology programs
- Schema therapy training centers
- Often offer reduced-fee services with trainees

Case Example 2: Marcus's Search Strategy

Marcus needed a schema therapist but felt overwhelmed by options. His systematic approach:

1. **Insurance check**: Got list of 20 covered providers
2. **Psychology Today cross-reference**: 5 listed schema therapy
3. **Consultation calls**: Scheduled 15-minute calls with all 5
4. **Questions asked**: Training, experience with perfectionism, approach
5. **Gut check**: Noted who he felt most comfortable with
6. **Decision**: Chose therapist with warm but structured style

"The calls were anxiety-provoking but worth it," Marcus reflected. "I could tell who understood schemas versus who just listed it as a keyword" [45].

What to Expect in Schema Therapy

Knowing what to expect reduces anxiety about starting therapy. Schema therapy typically follows a predictable structure:

Brief, Non-Intimidating Overview

Phase 1: Assessment and Education (Sessions 1-4)

- Discuss current problems and goals
- Explore childhood history gently
- Identify your main schemas
- Learn about schema therapy model
- Develop shared understanding

Phase 2: Change Strategies (Core of therapy)

- Cognitive techniques (examining evidence)
- Experiential techniques (imagery, chair work)
- Behavioral pattern-breaking
- Therapy relationship as lab for new patterns
- Homework between sessions

Phase 3: Integration (Final phase)

- Consolidate gains
- Prepare for future challenges

- Develop maintenance plan

- Process ending relationship

- Celebrate growth

Session Structure (Typical)

- Check-in about week and homework (10 min)

- Focus on specific issue or technique (30 min)

- Plan homework and next steps (10 min)

- Process session experience (10 min)

How It Builds on Your Self-Work

Your self-help work provides excellent foundation for therapy:

You Bring:

- Schema awareness

- Tried techniques

- Knowledge of triggers

- Questions and stuck points

- Motivation for change

Therapist Adds:

- Professional assessment

- Advanced techniques

- Trauma processing skills

- Relational healing

- Objective perspective

Together You Create:

- Deeper healing than either alone
- Faster progress
- Lasting change
- Corrective experiences
- New relational template

Case Example 3: Rosa's Therapy Journey

Rosa started therapy after a year of self-help work on her defectiveness schema. "I expected to start from scratch, but my therapist was impressed with my self-awareness. We skipped months of basic education because I already understood schemas."

Therapy added dimensions Rosa couldn't access alone:

- Imagery work to comfort her inner child
- Processing specific trauma memories safely
- Using the therapeutic relationship to test being "seen"
- EMDR for stuck trauma responses
- Group therapy to normalize her experience

"Self-help gave me the map," Rosa explained. "Therapy helped me actually travel the territory with a skilled guide" [46].

Continuing Your Journey

Schema healing is a marathon, not a sprint. Whether you continue with self-help, add professional support, or combine both, your journey continues.

Self-Help as Complement to Therapy

Many people combine approaches:

During Therapy:

- Continue daily practices
- Journal about sessions
- Practice homework assignments
- Read recommended books
- Join support groups

Between Therapy Phases:

- Some do intensive therapy, then self-help maintenance
- Others alternate periods of therapy and solo work
- Many return to therapy for "tune-ups" during life transitions

After Therapy:

- Maintain daily schema awareness
- Use tools learned in therapy
- Return if new schemas activate
- Become your own therapist

Long-Term Maintenance Strategies

Schema work is lifelong, but it gets easier:

Year 1-2: Intensive learning and practice

- Daily awareness needed
- Frequent tool use
- Regular setbacks
- Building new patterns

Year 3-5: Integration and solidifying

- More automatic healthy responses
- Quicker setback recovery
- Less daily effort needed
- Deeper self-compassion

Year 5+: Maintenance and growth

- Schemas whisper rather than shout
- Natural self-correction
- Helping others on journey
- Living from authentic self

Lifetime Practices:

- Annual schema check-ins
- Stress management for vulnerability
- Relationship pattern awareness
- Self-compassion as default
- Celebrating growth regularly

Your Ongoing Journey

Whether you continue solo or seek professional support, honor how far you've come. Reading this book, doing the exercises, facing your schemas—these take tremendous courage. You've started rewriting stories written in childhood, questioning beliefs that felt like truth, and choosing growth over familiar pain.

Schema work isn't about becoming someone new. It's about uncovering who you've always been beneath the protective layers. Your schemas served you once. Thank them for their protection, then choose which voices guide your future.

Some days, schemas will feel loud again. That's okay. You have tools now. You understand the game. Most importantly, you know you deserve healing, happiness, and healthy relationships. That knowledge alone changes everything.

Key Takeaways

- **Seeking therapy shows wisdom**, not weakness or failure
- **Multiple indicators suggest** when professional help would benefit your journey
- **Complex trauma typically requires** professional support for safe processing
- **Finding the right therapist** involves research, questions, and trusting your instincts
- **Schema therapy follows phases** from assessment through change to integration
- **Your self-help work** provides excellent foundation for therapy

- **Therapy adds dimensions** difficult to access through self-help alone

- **Combining approaches** often yields the best results

- **Long-term maintenance** gets easier as new patterns become automatic

- **Schema work is lifelong** but transforms from intensive work to gentle awareness

- **You deserve support** in whatever form helps you heal and grow

The Journey Continues

As you close this book, you're not ending your schema journey—you're beginning a new chapter. You have knowledge your younger self desperately needed. You have tools that actually work. You have permission to heal at your own pace, in your own way.

Some of you will take these tools and transform your lives through dedicated self-practice. Others will use this book as a stepping stone to professional help. Many will weave between both approaches as life unfolds. All paths are valid. All lead toward the same destination: a life guided by choice rather than compulsion, love rather than fear, truth rather than outdated stories.

Your schemas might never completely disappear. But they can become like old scars—reminders of what you've survived rather than directors of your future. In their place, new beliefs can grow: I am enough. I belong here. I deserve love. I can trust wisely. I am capable. These aren't just affirmations anymore. With practice, patience, and compassion, they become lived truth.

The child who developed these schemas did their best with impossible situations. Now the adult you've become can offer what that child always needed: understanding, safety, and unconditional love. That's the ultimate schema therapy—becoming the healing presence your younger self was looking for.

Welcome to the rest of your life. It's yours to write.

Appendix A: Quick Reference Guides

A therapist once told me that healing happens in the moments when you need help most but can't access your full toolkit. "That's why I give my clients cheat sheets," she said, sliding a laminated card across her desk. "When your schema is screaming and you can't remember Chapter 5, you need something simple, immediate, and effective." This appendix is your collection of cheat sheets—quick references for those moments when schemas activate and you need help fast. Keep these pages bookmarked, photograph them for your phone, or copy the parts most relevant to you. Think of them as emergency supplies for your psychological first aid kit.

All 18 Schemas Quick Description and Coping Strategies

Each schema gets a two-page spread here—enough to remind you what you're dealing with and how to respond, but brief enough to use during activation.

1. Abandonment/Instability Schema

Quick Description: The deep fear that people you care about will leave, die, or emotionally abandon you. You expect instability in close relationships.

How It Shows Up:

- Panic when partner doesn't text back quickly

- Clinging or pushing people away preemptively

- Interpreting normal distance as rejection

- Constantly seeking reassurance

Emergency Coping Strategies:

- **Immediate**: Hand on heart, say "This feeling is familiar, not factual"

- **5-Minute**: Call/text a stable friend who's been in your life 2+ years

- **When Calmer**: Write evidence of people who've stayed

- **Daily Practice**: Morning affirmation: "I am whole with or without others"

- **Behavioral Test**: Wait 10 extra minutes before seeking reassurance

2. Mistrust/Abuse Schema

Quick Description: The expectation that others will hurt, abuse, humiliate, cheat, lie, manipulate, or take advantage of you.

How It Shows Up:

- Hypervigilance about others' motives

- Testing people's loyalty repeatedly

- Difficulty accepting kindness at face value

- Keeping emotional walls up

Emergency Coping Strategies:

- **Immediate**: Notice physical tension, consciously relax jaw and shoulders

- **5-Minute**: List three people who've been trustworthy

- **When Calmer**: Separate past betrayals from present person

- **Daily Practice**: Notice one kind act without analyzing motives

- **Behavioral Test**: Accept help without investigating ulterior motives

3. Emotional Deprivation Schema

Quick Description: The belief that your need for emotional support, nurturing, empathy, and protection will never be adequately met by others.

How It Shows Up:

- Feeling alone even with others

- Not expressing emotional needs

- Believing no one truly understands you

- Settling for crumbs of affection

Emergency Coping Strategies:

- **Immediate**: Give yourself the understanding you seek

- **5-Minute**: Write what you need to hear, then read it aloud

- **When Calmer**: Ask one person for specific emotional support

- **Daily Practice**: Notice when emotional needs ARE met, however small

- **Behavioral Test**: Express one feeling to someone safe

4. Defectiveness/Shame Schema

Quick Description: The feeling that you're defective, bad, unwanted, inferior, or unlovable in important respects.

How It Shows Up:

- Hiding authentic self
- Extreme sensitivity to criticism
- Believing compliments are lies or politeness
- Fear of being "found out"

Emergency Coping Strategies:

- **Immediate:** "I am human and therefore imperfect and worthy"
- **5-Minute:** List three things you like about yourself
- **When Calmer:** Share something genuine with trusted person
- **Daily Practice:** Mirror work - one kind thing to reflection daily
- **Behavioral Test:** Let someone see you without "performing"

5. Social Isolation/Alienation Schema

Quick Description: The feeling that you're isolated from the world, different from others, and/or not part of any group or community.

How It Shows Up:

- Feeling like an outsider everywhere
- Believing you don't belong
- Avoiding group situations
- Emphasizing differences over similarities

Emergency Coping Strategies:

- **Immediate:** "Different doesn't mean defective"

- **5-Minute:** Recall one moment of belonging

- **When Calmer:** List communities where you have membership

- **Daily Practice:** Notice one similarity with someone daily

- **Behavioral Test:** Attend one group activity this week

6. Dependence/Incompetence Schema

Quick Description: The belief that you're unable to handle everyday responsibilities competently without considerable help from others.

How It Shows Up:

- Avoiding new challenges

- Constant advice-seeking for minor decisions

- Believing others are more capable

- Learned helplessness patterns

Emergency Coping Strategies:

- **Immediate:** "I can figure this out one step at a time"

- **5-Minute:** List three things you've handled independently

- **When Calmer:** Break overwhelming task into tiny steps

- **Daily Practice**: Make one decision without consulting anyone
- **Behavioral Test**: Try something new without asking for help first

7. Vulnerability to Harm/Illness Schema

Quick Description: Exaggerated fear that imminent catastrophe will strike at any time and that you'll be unable to prevent it.

How It Shows Up:

- Constant worry about disasters
- Excessive health anxiety
- Avoiding normal activities due to danger fears
- Catastrophic thinking patterns

Emergency Coping Strategies:

- **Immediate**: "I am safe in this moment"
- **5-Minute**: Ground with 5-4-3-2-1 senses technique
- **When Calmer**: Calculate actual versus feared probability
- **Daily Practice**: Notice when feared outcomes don't happen
- **Behavioral Test**: Do one "risky" but normal activity

8. Enmeshment/Undeveloped Self Schema

Quick Description: Excessive emotional involvement with important others at the expense of full individuation or normal social development.

How It Shows Up:

- Not knowing your own preferences

- Feeling guilty for independence

- Taking on others' emotions as your own

- No clear personal boundaries

Emergency Coping Strategies:

- **Immediate**: "I am a separate person with valid needs"

- **5-Minute**: List three preferences that differ from loved ones

- **When Calmer**: Practice saying "I think/feel" statements

- **Daily Practice**: Make one choice based solely on your preference

- **Behavioral Test**: Disagree gently about something minor

9. Failure Schema

Quick Description: The belief that you have failed, will inevitably fail, or are fundamentally inadequate in areas of achievement.

How It Shows Up:

- Avoiding challenges to prevent failure

- Dismissing successes as luck

- Comparing yourself negatively to others

- Giving up quickly when things get hard

Emergency Coping Strategies:

- **Immediate**: "Mistakes are information, not identity"
- **5-Minute**: Write three past successes, however small
- **When Calmer**: Reframe recent "failure" as learning
- **Daily Practice**: Celebrate one effort regardless of outcome
- **Behavioral Test**: Try something with 50% success chance

10. Entitlement/Grandiosity Schema

Quick Description: The belief that you're superior to others, entitled to special rights, or not bound by normal social rules.

How It Shows Up:

- Difficulty with rules or limits
- Expecting special treatment
- Low empathy for others' needs
- Rage when not given priority

Emergency Coping Strategies:

- **Immediate**: "Everyone's needs matter, including mine"
- **5-Minute**: Consider situation from others' perspective
- **When Calmer**: List ways others are special too
- **Daily Practice**: Follow one rule you usually bend

- **Behavioral Test**: Wait your turn without complaint

11. Insufficient Self-Control/Self-Discipline Schema

Quick Description: Difficulty exercising self-control and frustration tolerance to achieve goals or restrain excessive emotions/impulses.

How It Shows Up:

- Acting on immediate impulses
- Difficulty with routine or structure
- Avoiding discomfort at all costs
- Pattern of starting but not finishing

Emergency Coping Strategies:

- **Immediate**: "I can pause between impulse and action"
- **5-Minute**: Do one small disciplined act (make bed, etc.)
- **When Calmer**: Plan one structure for tomorrow
- **Daily Practice**: Build one tiny consistent habit
- **Behavioral Test**: Delay one gratification by 10 minutes

12. Subjugation Schema

Quick Description: Excessive surrendering of control to others to avoid anger, retaliation, or abandonment.

How It Shows Up:

- Chronically putting others first

- Difficulty saying no

- Suppressing own needs/opinions

- Resentment building under compliance

Emergency Coping Strategies:

- **Immediate:** "My needs are as valid as others'"

- **5-Minute:** Write what YOU want in this situation

- **When Calmer:** Practice saying no to mirror

- **Daily Practice:** Express one preference daily

- **Behavioral Test:** Say no to one small request

13. Self-Sacrifice Schema

Quick Description: Excessive focus on meeting others' needs at the expense of your own gratification.

How It Shows Up:

- Guilt when focusing on self

- Pride in never needing anything

- Burnout from giving too much

- Others depending on your sacrifice

Emergency Coping Strategies:

- **Immediate:** "Self-care enables care for others"

- **5-Minute:** Do one kind thing for yourself

- **When Calmer:** Schedule personal time like appointment

- **Daily Practice:** Meet one of your needs before others'

- **Behavioral Test**: Accept help when offered

14. Approval-Seeking/Recognition-Seeking Schema

Quick Description: Excessive emphasis on gaining approval, recognition, or attention from others.

How It Shows Up:

- Changing behavior based on audience
- Devastation from criticism
- Constant need for validation
- Loss of authentic self

Emergency Coping Strategies:

- **Immediate**: "I approve of myself in this moment"
- **5-Minute**: List what YOU like about recent action
- **When Calmer**: Journal about your values
- **Daily Practice**: Make one choice without sharing it
- **Behavioral Test**: Post/say something without checking responses

15. Negativity/Pessimism Schema

Quick Description: Pervasive focus on negative aspects of life while minimizing positive aspects.

How It Shows Up:

- Expecting worst outcomes
- Dismissing good news as temporary
- "Yes, but..." thinking patterns

- Difficulty enjoying positive moments

Emergency Coping Strategies:

- **Immediate:** "Good and bad both exist"
- **5-Minute:** Force-list three current positives
- **When Calmer:** Write balanced view of situation
- **Daily Practice:** Gratitude practice (three specific items)
- **Behavioral Test:** Share one optimistic thought

16. Emotional Inhibition Schema

Quick Description: Excessive inhibition of spontaneous emotions, actions, or communication to avoid disapproval or shame.

How It Shows Up:

- Difficulty expressing feelings
- Appearing cold or controlled
- Fear of losing control if emotional
- Physical tension from suppression

Emergency Coping Strategies:

- **Immediate:** "Feelings are human and safe"
- **5-Minute:** Name emotions in body privately
- **When Calmer:** Express feeling through art/writing
- **Daily Practice:** Share one small emotion daily
- **Behavioral Test:** Show enthusiasm about something

17. Unrelenting Standards/Hypercriticalness Schema

Quick Description: The belief that you must meet very high internalized standards to avoid criticism.

How It Shows Up:

- Perfectionism paralyzing action
- Never feeling good enough
- Criticizing self and others harshly
- Burnout from overworking

Emergency Coping Strategies:

- **Immediate**: "Good enough is good enough"
- **5-Minute**: List what's already sufficient
- **When Calmer**: Set "minimum viable" standard
- **Daily Practice**: Leave one thing imperfect
- **Behavioral Test**: Submit B+ work instead of A+

18. Punitiveness Schema

Quick Description: The belief that people should be harshly punished for mistakes.

How It Shows Up:

- Harsh self-criticism for errors
- Difficulty forgiving self or others
- Black-and-white thinking about mistakes
- Rage at imperfection

Emergency Coping Strategies:

- **Immediate**: "Mistakes deserve compassion"
- **5-Minute**: Consider mistake's actual impact
- **When Calmer**: Write self-forgiveness letter
- **Daily Practice**: Find lesson instead of punishment
- **Behavioral Test**: Respond gently to one mistake

Emergency Coping Menu by Emotion

When schemas activate, you often can't think clearly enough to remember what helps. This menu organizes coping strategies by the emotion you're feeling.

When You Feel Panicked/Terrified

- **Breathe**: 4-7-8 breathing (in for 4, hold for 7, out for 8)
- **Ground**: Name 5 things you see, 4 you hear, 3 you touch, 2 you smell, 1 you taste
- **Move**: Walk, shake out limbs, do jumping jacks
- **Cool**: Splash cold water on face, hold ice cube
- **Affirm**: "This feeling will pass. I am safe right now."

When You Feel Worthless/Ashamed

- **Comfort**: Hand on heart, self-hug, soft blanket
- **Counter**: Read saved compliments or achievements
- **Connect**: Text someone who loves you
- **Create**: Draw, write, or make something imperfect
- **Affirm**: "I am worthy of love and respect"

When You Feel Angry/Rageful

- **Release**: Hit pillows, scream in car, tear paper
- **Move**: Run, dance aggressively, do pushups
- **Cool**: Cold shower, ice on temples
- **Write**: Angry letter you won't send
- **Affirm**: "Anger is information. I can respond wisely."

When You Feel Hopeless/Despairing

- **Light**: Sit in sunlight or bright light
- **Small**: Do one tiny positive action
- **Remember**: Read past journal entries showing change
- **Connect**: Call crisis line if needed
- **Affirm**: "This darkness is temporary. Dawn comes."

When You Feel Lonely/Abandoned

- **Reach**: Text three people, even just "Hi"
- **Comfort**: Hug pillow, pet animal, warm bath
- **Watch**: Comforting show with familiar characters
- **Visit**: Go where people are (coffee shop, library)
- **Affirm**: "I belong in this world. Connection is possible."

When You Feel Anxious/Worried

- **Breathe**: Square breathing (4 counts each: in, hold, out, hold)
- **Move**: Gentle yoga, walk, stretch

- **Focus**: One task requiring concentration

- **Limit**: No catastrophic news or social media

- **Affirm**: "I can handle whatever comes"

Schema Trigger Tracker

Use this format to track patterns over time:

Date: _____ Time: _____ Trigger Event:
_____ Schema

Activated: _____ Emotion

Intensity (1-10): _____ Body

Sensations: _____

Automatic Thoughts: _____

How I Responded: _____

What Helped: _____

What Didn't Help: _____

Recovery Time: _____

Learning for Next Time: _____

Appendix B: Extended Exercises

Some healing work requires more space and depth than daily practices allow. These extended exercises are for when you have time and emotional bandwidth for deeper exploration. Use them during calm periods, not during crisis. Consider having support available—a trusted friend, therapist, or support group—as these exercises can bring up strong emotions.

Advanced Imagery Scripts

These scripts go beyond basic inner child work to facilitate deeper healing experiences.

The Schema Timeline Journey

Purpose: To understand how your schema developed and identify points of resilience

Time Needed: 45-60 minutes

Preparation:

- Quiet, private space

- Journal nearby

- Comfort items available

- Support person on standby if needed

Script:

Settle into a comfortable position. Close your eyes and take five deep breaths, allowing your body to relax more with each exhale.

In your mind's eye, imagine a long hallway. This hallway represents your life timeline. You're standing at a door marked "Present." Looking down the hallway, you see other doors, each representing a different age in your life.

Begin walking slowly down this hallway, moving backward through time. Notice doors marked with ages—last year, five years ago, ten years ago. You're safe here; you're an observer with all your adult resources.

Continue until you find a door that feels significant to your schema. Maybe it glows differently or draws your attention. This might be when your schema first formed or strongly activated.

Approach this door. Before opening it, remind yourself: "I am visiting this memory with compassion and adult wisdom. I can leave anytime."

Open the door and observe the scene. See your younger self there. Notice:

- How old are they?

- What's happening?

- What are they feeling?

- What do they need?

Without changing the past event, you can offer your younger self what they need. Maybe it's:

- Words of comfort

- A protective presence

- Truth about the situation

- Promise of survival

Stay as long as feels right. When ready, invite your younger self to leave with you. Some may come immediately; others need more time. That's okay.

Walk back down the hallway together, stopping at doors marking positive memories or moments of strength. Show your younger self: "See? We made it. We survived. We even had joy."

Return to the present door. Thank your younger self for their courage. Let them know they can stay with you in the present, where it's safe.

Take five deep breaths. Feel your body in the chair. When ready, open your eyes.

After the Exercise:

- Journal immediately about what you experienced

- Be extra gentle with yourself for 24 hours

- Share with support person if helpful

- Notice any shifts in how you relate to your schema

The Compassionate Parent Visualization

Purpose: To provide yourself with the parenting you needed but didn't receive

Time Needed: 30 minutes

Script:

Close your eyes and imagine yourself in a beautiful, safe space—perhaps a cozy room with a fireplace or a peaceful garden. This is your healing space.

Now imagine the ideal parent figure approaching. This might be:

- A wiser version of yourself
- An archetypal figure (wise woman, protective father)
- A composite of various caring figures
- Pure loving energy in human form

This compassionate parent radiates the exact qualities you needed:

- Unconditional love
- Consistent presence
- Appropriate protection
- Encouragement
- Understanding

They sit near you and say, "I see you. I see all of you—your struggles, your pain, your incredible strength. I'm here now."

Allow yourself to receive what they offer:

- If you needed protection, feel them standing guard
- If you needed encouragement, hear their belief in you
- If you needed understanding, feel deeply seen
- If you needed consistency, know they'll always be available

You might want to:

- Tell them about your pain

- Ask questions you've always had

- Simply sit in their presence

- Receive a hug if wanted

Stay in this connection as long as needed. Before leaving, your compassionate parent figure says, "I'm not just here now. I'm always available. When your schema activates, call on me. I'll remind you of your worth."

Slowly return to the room. Know you can revisit this figure anytime.

Relationship Dialogue Practices

These exercises help you practice new ways of relating before trying them in real relationships.

The Empty Chair Technique

Purpose: To practice difficult conversations and work through relationship patterns

Setup:

- Two chairs facing each other

- Privacy to speak aloud

- Specific person/situation in mind

Process:

1. **Identify the Conversation:** Choose a relationship where schemas activate strongly

2. **Set the Scene:** One chair is you, other is the person

3. **Speak Your Truth:** Sit in your chair and say what you've needed to express

4. **Switch Chairs**: Physically move to other chair, embody other person

5. **Respond as Them**: Let them speak through you

6. **Continue Dialogue**: Keep switching chairs as conversation unfolds

7. **Find Resolution**: Not agreement, but understanding

What to Express:

- How their behavior triggers your schema

- What you needed but didn't get

- Your boundaries going forward

- Appreciation for any positives

- Your commitment to your own healing

The Relationship Repair Script

Purpose: To heal a specific relationship moment that reinforced your schema

Process:

1. **Choose a Moment**: Select specific interaction that strengthened your schema

2. **Write the Original**: Script exactly what was said/done

3. **Identify Schema Message**: What did your schema conclude?

4. **Rewrite with Health**: How could it have gone differently?

5. **Practice New Version**: Read aloud, embody the feeling

6. **Integration**: Notice how the new version feels in your body

Example:

Original: You (age 8): "Mom, look at my drawing!" Mom: "Not now, I'm busy. Stop bothering me." Schema message: "My needs are bothersome"

Rewritten: You (age 8): "Mom, look at my drawing!" Mom: "I can see this is important to you. Let me finish this one thing and then I want to see it." New message: "My needs matter and will be attended to"

Monthly Progress Review Template

Regular reviews help you see progress that daily life obscures.

Monthly Schema Health Check-In

Date: _____

Overall Schema Activity This Month: Rate each of your top 3 schemas (1-10, where 10 is highly active):

1. _____: ____/10 (Last month: ____/10)

2. _____: ____/10 (Last month: ____/10)

3. _____: ____/10 (Last month: ____/10)

Wins and Progress:

- Situations handled differently:

   _____

- New behaviors tried:

  _____

- Moments of self-compassion:

  _____

- Relationship improvements:

  _____

Challenges and Setbacks:

- Difficult triggers:

  _____

- Setback situations:

  _____

- What helped recovery:

  _____

Patterns Noticed:

- Times schemas most active:

  _____

- Times schemas quieter:

  _____

- Environmental factors:

  _____

Tools and Techniques:

- Most helpful this month:

  _____

- Least helpful:

  _____

- Want to try next month:

  _____

Relationship Patterns:

- Schema dynamics noticed:

  _____

- Progress in relationships:

  _____

- Areas for attention:

  _____

Self-Care and Support:

- Self-care practices maintained:

  _____

- Support utilized:

  _____

- Additional support needed:

  _____

Next Month's Focus:

- Primary goal:

  _____

- Specific experiments planned:

  _____

- Support arrangements:

  _____

Compassionate Message to Myself:

One Thing I'm Proud Of:

Appendix C: Recommended Resources

Your schema healing journey doesn't end with this book. Here are carefully selected resources to support your continued growth.

Books for Deeper Exploration

Core Schema Therapy Books:

"Reinventing Your Life" by Jeffrey Young and Janet Klosko

- The foundational self-help book on schemas

- Detailed questionnaires and exercises

- Case examples for each schema

"Schema Therapy: A Practitioner's Guide" by Jeffrey Young, Janet Klosko, and Marjorie Weishaar

- Professional text but accessible to motivated readers

- Deeper understanding of schema theory

- Advanced techniques explained

"Breaking Negative Thinking Patterns" by Gitta Jacob and Hannie van Genderen

- Practical workbook format

- Step-by-step exercises

- Focus on changing thought patterns

Related Therapeutic Approaches:

"Self-Compassion" by Kristin Neff

- Essential for schema healing journey

- Research-based compassion practices

- Addresses self-criticism directly

"The Body Keeps the Score" by Bessel van der Kolk

- Understanding trauma's impact on schemas

- Body-based healing approaches

- Comprehensive trauma resource

"Attached" by Amir Levine and Rachel Heller

- Understanding attachment styles

- How schemas affect relationships

- Practical relationship guidance

For Specific Issues:

"Complex PTSD" by Pete Walker

- For schemas rooted in childhood trauma

- Practical recovery strategies

- Compassionate approach

"The Emotionally Absent Mother" by Jasmin Lee Cori

- For emotional deprivation schemas

- Healing mother wounds

- Building self-nurturing skills

Apps for Meditation and Mood Tracking

Meditation Apps with Schema-Relevant Content:

Insight Timer

- Free meditation library
- Search "inner child" or "self-compassion"
- Community support features
- Progress tracking

Headspace

- Structured meditation courses
- "Managing Anxiety" pack helps with abandonment fears
- "Self-esteem" course for defectiveness schemas
- Sleep stories for vulnerability schemas

Calm

- Daily calm sessions
- Anxiety release programs
- Sleep stories and music
- Panic attack support

Ten Percent Happier

- Skeptic-friendly approach
- Courses on difficult emotions
- Direct, practical style
- Good for emotional inhibition schemas

Mood Tracking Apps:

Daylio

- Quick daily mood tracking
- Identifies patterns over time
- Correlates activities with moods
- No typing required

eMoods

- Detailed mood tracking
- Medication tracking if relevant
- PDF reports for therapy
- Pattern identification

Sanvello

- Mood tracking plus coping tools
- Guided journeys for specific issues
- Community support
- Some insurance coverage

DBT Coach

- Dialectical behavior therapy skills
- Emotion regulation tools
- Distress tolerance techniques
- Good for self-control schemas

Online Communities and Support

Moderated Forums:

Schema Therapy Forum (Psychology Today)

- Professional moderation
- Schema-specific discussions
- Success stories and support

Reddit Communities:

- r/SchemaTherapy - Growing community
- r/CPTSD - For trauma-related schemas
- r/DecidingToBeBetter - General growth support
- Read rules, avoid comparing traumas

Facebook Groups (Search for):

- "Schema Therapy Support Group"
- "Healing Your Inner Child"
- Specific schema-focused groups
- Verify active moderation

Important Notes for Online Support:

- Verify group rules and moderation
- Protect your privacy
- Take what helps, leave the rest
- Online support supplements, doesn't replace therapy
- Be cautious of unqualified advice

Professional Organization Directories

International Society of Schema Therapy (ISST)

- Website: www.schematherapy.org
- Global therapist directory
- Training standards information
- Research updates

American Psychological Association

- Website: www.apa.org
- Psychologist locator tool
- Verification of credentials
- Consumer resources

National Association of Social Workers

- Website: www.socialworkers.org
- Social worker directory
- Specialty area searches
- Insurance information

International Centre for Excellence in EFT

- Website: www.iceeft.com
- For relationship schema work
- Emotionally focused therapy
- Couple therapy specialists

EMDRIA (EMDR International Association)

- Website: www.emdria.org
- For trauma-related schemas

- Certified practitioner directory
- Training standards

Crisis Resources

If schemas trigger crisis:

National Suicide Prevention Lifeline: 988 (US) **Crisis Text Line**: Text HOME to 741741 **International Hotlines**: findahelpline.com

Creating Your Resource Library

You don't need all these resources. Start with:

1. One additional schema book
2. One meditation app
3. One mood tracking method
4. Bookmarked therapist directories

Build your library slowly, based on what actually helps rather than what seems impressive. Quality engagement with few resources beats surface skimming of many.

Your Toolkit for Life

These appendices are your reference manual for the ongoing journey of schema healing. The quick guides help during activation. The extended exercises deepen your practice. The resources connect you with larger healing communities.

Schema work is like tending a garden. Some days you plant new seeds (trying new behaviors). Other days you pull weeds (catching schema activation). Sometimes you simply water what's already growing (maintaining progress). And occasionally, you step back to appreciate how far your garden has come.

Keep these tools close. Use what works. Adapt what doesn't. Trust your instincts about what you need when. Most importantly, be patient with yourself. You're rewriting stories written in childhood, healing wounds that run deep, and creating new patterns for generations to come. That's heroic work, even when it feels ordinary.

Your schemas may always whisper, but they no longer have to shout. With these tools, consistent practice, and boundless self-compassion, you're writing a new story—one where you're not just surviving your schemas, but thriving beyond them.

Reference

[1] Young, J. E., Klosko, J. S., & Weishaar, M. E. (2003). Schema therapy: A practitioner's guide. Guilford Press.

[2] Young, J. E. (1999). Cognitive therapy for personality disorders: A schema-focused approach (3rd ed.). Professional Resource Press.

[3] Arntz, A., & van Genderen, H. (2009). Schema therapy for borderline personality disorder. Wiley-Blackwell.

[4] Rafaeli, E., Bernstein, D. P., & Young, J. (2011). Schema therapy: Distinctive features. Routledge.

[5] Lockwood, G., & Shaw, I. (2012). Schema therapy for eating disorders: A case illustration. In M. van Vreeswijk, J. Broersen, & M. Nadort (Eds.), The Wiley-Blackwell handbook of schema therapy (pp. 145-172). John Wiley & Sons.

[6] Farrell, J. M., & Shaw, I. A. (2012). Group schema therapy for borderline personality disorder: A step-by-step treatment manual with patient workbook. Wiley-Blackwell.

[7] Beck, A. T., Freeman, A., & Davis, D. D. (2004). Cognitive therapy of personality disorders (2nd ed.). Guilford Press.

[8] Roediger, E. (2012). Schema therapy for avoidant personality disorder. In M. van Vreeswijk, J. Broersen, & M. Nadort (Eds.), The Wiley-Blackwell handbook of schema therapy (pp. 197-214). John Wiley & Sons.

[9] van der Kolk, B. A. (2014). The body keeps the score: Brain, mind, and body in the healing of trauma. Viking.

[10] Greenberg, L. S. (2002). Emotion-focused therapy: Coaching clients to work through their feelings. American Psychological Association.

[11] Teasdale, J. D., & Barnard, P. J. (1993). Affect, cognition, and change: Re-modelling depressive thought. Lawrence Erlbaum Associates.

[12] Simpson, S. G., Morrow, E., van Vreeswijk, M., & Reid, C. (2010). Group schema therapy for eating disorders: A pilot study. Frontiers in Psychology, 1, 182.

[13] Jacob, G. A., & Arntz, A. (2013). Schema therapy for personality disorders—A review. International Journal of Cognitive Therapy, 6(2), 171-185.

[14] Bamelis, L. L., Evers, S. M., Spinhoven, P., & Arntz, A. (2014). Results of a multicenter randomized controlled trial of the clinical effectiveness of schema therapy for personality disorders. American Journal of Psychiatry, 171(3), 305-322.

[15] Dweck, C. S. (2013). Social development. In P. D. Zelazo (Ed.), The Oxford handbook of developmental psychology (Vol. 2, pp. 167-190). Oxford University Press.

[16] Bowlby, J. (1988). A secure base: Parent-child attachment and healthy human development. Basic Books.

[17] Siegel, D. J., & Hartzell, M. (2003). Parenting from the inside out: How a deeper self-understanding can help you raise children who thrive. Jeremy P. Tarcher/Penguin.

[18] Burns, D. D. (1980). Feeling good: The new mood therapy. William Morrow and Company.

[19] Main, M., & Solomon, J. (1986). Discovery of an insecure-disorganized/disoriented attachment pattern. In T. B. Brazelton & M. W. Yogman (Eds.), Affective development in infancy (pp. 95-124). Ablex Publishing.

[20] Miller, A. (1981). The drama of the gifted child: The search for the true self. Basic Books.

[21] Herman, J. L. (1992). Trauma and recovery: The aftermath of violence—from domestic abuse to political terror. Basic Books.

[22] Siegel, D. J. (2012). The developing mind: How relationships and the brain interact to shape who we are (2nd ed.). Guilford Press.

[23] Shapiro, F. (2001). Eye movement desensitization and reprocessing (EMDR): Basic principles, protocols, and procedures (2nd ed.). Guilford Press.

[24] Malchiodi, C. A. (2012). Art therapy and the brain. In C. A. Malchiodi (Ed.), Handbook of art therapy (2nd ed., pp. 17-26). Guilford Press.

[25] Johnson, S. M. (1994). Character styles. W. W. Norton & Company.

[26] Gilbert, P. (2009). The compassionate mind: A new approach to life's challenges. New Harbinger Publications.

[27] Parnell, L. (2013). Attachment-focused EMDR: Healing relational trauma. W. W. Norton & Company.

[28] Bennett-Levy, J., Butler, G., Fennell, M., Hackmann, A., Mueller, M., & Westbrook, D. (2004). Oxford guide to behavioural experiments in cognitive therapy. Oxford University Press.

[29] Padesky, C. A. (1994). Schema change processes in cognitive therapy. Clinical Psychology & Psychotherapy, 1(5), 267-278.

[30] Wells, A. (1997). Cognitive therapy of anxiety disorders: A practice manual and conceptual guide. John Wiley & Sons.

[31] Leahy, R. L. (2003). Cognitive therapy techniques: A practitioner's guide. Guilford Press.

[32] Wood, J. V., Perunovic, W. Q. E., & Lee, J. W. (2009). Positive self-statements: Power for some, peril for others. Psychological Science, 20(7), 860-866.

[33] Kearney, D. J., Malte, C. A., McManus, C., Martinez, M. E., Felleman, B., & Simpson, T. L. (2013). Loving-kindness meditation for posttraumatic stress disorder: A pilot study. Journal of Traumatic Stress, 26(4), 426-434.

[34] Linehan, M. M. (2014). DBT Skills Training Manual (2nd ed.). Guilford Press.

[35] Pennebaker, J. W. (1997). Writing about emotional experiences as a therapeutic process. Psychological Science, 8(3), 162-166.

[36] Hazan, C., & Shaver, P. (1987). Romantic love conceptualized as an attachment process. Journal of Personality and Social Psychology, 52(3), 511-524.

[37] Johnson, S. M. (2019). Attachment theory in practice: Emotionally focused therapy (EFT) with individuals, couples, and families. Guilford Press.

[38] Geller, S. M., & Greenberg, L. S. (2012). Therapeutic presence: A mindful approach to effective therapy. American Psychological Association.

[39] Doidge, N. (2007). The brain that changes itself: Stories of personal triumph from the frontiers of brain science. Viking.

[40] Porges, S. W. (2011). The polyvagal theory: Neurophysiological foundations of emotions, attachment, communication, and self-regulation. W. W. Norton & Company.

[41] Neff, K. D. (2011). Self-compassion: The proven power of being kind to yourself. William Morrow.

[42] Germer, C. K. (2009). The mindful path to self-compassion: Freeing yourself from destructive thoughts and emotions. Guilford Press.

[43] Hayes, S. C., Strosahl, K. D., & Wilson, K. G. (2012). Acceptance and commitment therapy: The process and practice of mindful change (2nd ed.). Guilford Press.

[44] Tatkin, S. (2012). Wired for love: How understanding your partner's brain and attachment style can help you defuse conflict and build a secure relationship. New Harbinger Publications.

[45] Cozolino, L. (2010). The neuroscience of psychotherapy: Healing the social brain (2nd ed.). W. W. Norton & Company.

[46] Levine, P. A. (2010). In an unspoken voice: How the body releases trauma and restores goodness. North Atlantic Books.